Primary Immunodeficiency Disorders

Editor

ANTHONY MONTANARO

IMMUNOLOGY AND ALLERGY CLINICS OF NORTH AMERICA

www.immunology.theclinics.com

November 2015 • Volume 35 • Number 4

ELSEVIER

1600 John F. Kennedy Boulevard • Suite 1800 • Philadelphia, Pennsylvania, 19103-2899
http://www.theclinics.com

IMMUNOLOGY AND ALLERGY CLINICS OF NORTH AMERICA Volume 35, Number 4
November 2015 ISSN 0889-8561, ISBN-13: 978-0-323-41334-3
Editor: Jessica McCool
Developmental Editor: Kristen Helm

Immunology and Allergy Clinics of North America (ISSN 0889–8561) is published quarterly by Elsevier Inc., 360 Park Avenue South, New York, NY 10010-1710. Months of issue are February, May, August, and November. Periodicals postage paid at New York, NY and additional mailing offices. Subscription prices are $320.00 per year for US individuals, $454.00 per year for US institutions, $150.00 per year for US students and residents, $395.00 per year for Canadian individuals, $220.00 per year for Canadian students, $577.00 per year for Canadian institutions, $445.00 per year for international individuals, $577.00 per year for international institutions, $220.00 per year for international students. To receive student/resident rate, orders must be accompanied by name of affiliated institution, date of term, and the *signature* of program/residency coordinator on institution letterhead. Orders will be billed at individual rate until proof of status is received. Foreign air speed delivery is included in all *Clinics* subscription prices. All prices are subject to change without notice. **POSTMASTER**: Send address changes to *Immunology and Allergy Clinics of North America,* Elsevier Health Sciences Division, Subscription Customer Service, 3251 Riverport Lane, Maryland Heights, MO 63043. **Customer Service: 1-800-654-2452 (U.S. and Canada); 314-447-8871 (outside U.S. and Canada). Fax: 314-447-8029. E-mail: journalscustomerservice-usa@elsevier.com (for print support); journalsonlinesupport-usa@elsevier.com (for online support).**

Reprints. For copies of 100 or more, of articles in this publication, please contact the Commercial Reprints Department, Elsevier Inc., 360 Park Avenue South, New York, New York 10010-1710. Tel. 212-633-3874, Fax: 212-633-3820, E-mail: reprints@elsevier.com.

Immunology and Allergy Clinics of North America is covered in MEDLINE/PubMed (Index Medicus), Current Contents/Life Sciences, Science Citation Index, ISI/BIOMED, Chemical Abstracts, and EMBASE/Excerpta Medica.

Contributors

EDITOR

ANTHONY MONTANARO, MD
Chief, Division of Allergy and Immunology, Oregon Health and Science University, Portland, Oregon

AUTHORS

JORDAN K. ABBOTT, MA, MD
Division of Allergy and Immunology, Department of Pediatrics, National Jewish Health, Denver, Colorado

MARK BALLOW, MD
Professor, Division of Allergy and Immunology, Department of Pediatrics, University of South Florida, Saint Petersburg, Florida

LAURI BURROUGHS, MD
Seattle Children's Hospital; Assistant Professor, Pediatrics, Bone Marrow Transplant, University of Washington School of Medicine; Director, Non-Malignant Transplant Program, Fred Hutchinson Cancer Research Center, Seattle, Washington

SANNY K. CHAN, MD, PhD
Assistant Professor, Division of Allergy and Immunology, Department of Pediatrics, National Jewish Health, Denver, Colorado

IVAN K. CHINN, MD
Assistant Professor of Pediatrics, Section of Immunology, Allergy, and Rheumatology, Department of Pediatrics, Texas Children's Hospital, Baylor College of Medicine, Houston, Texas

VICTORIA R. DIMITRIADES, MD
Assistant Professor, Section of Allergy Immunology, Department of Pediatrics, Louisiana State University Health Sciences Center, Jeffrey Modell Center for Primary Immunodeficiencies, New Orleans, Louisiana

CHITRA DINAKAR, MD
Division of Allergy, Asthma and Immunology, Department of Pediatrics, Children's Mercy Hospital, University of Missouri-Kansas City, Kansas City, Missouri

ERWIN W. GELFAND, MD
Professor, Division of Allergy and Immunology, Department of Pediatrics, National Jewish Health, Denver, Colorado

DAVID HAGIN, MD, PhD
Senior Fellow, Allergy/Immunology, Seattle Children's Hospital; University of Washington School of Medicine; Seattle Children's Research Institute, Seattle, Washington

VIVIAN P. HERNANDEZ-TRUJILLO, MD
Director, Division of Allergy and Immunology, Department of Pediatrics, Nicklaus Children's Hospital; Associate Clinical Professor, Herbert Wertheim School of Medicine, Florida International University, Miami, Florida

STEPHANIE NONAS, MD
Assistant Professor of Medicine, Division of Pulmonary and Critical Care Medicine, Medical Director of Respiratory Care, Oregon Health and Science University, Portland, Oregon

NIKITA RAJE, MD
Division of Allergy, Asthma and Immunology, Department of Pediatrics, Children's Mercy Hospital, University of Missouri-Kansas City, Kansas City, Missouri

MARYAM SAIFI, MD
Division of Allergy and Immunology, Department of Internal Medicine, UT Southwestern Medical Center, Dallas, Texas

WILLIAM T. SHEARER, MD, PhD
Section of Immunology, Allergy, and Rheumatology, Department of Pediatrics, Texas Children's Hospital, Baylor College of Medicine, Houston, Texas

RICARDO U. SORENSEN, MD
Professor and Chair, Section of Allergy Immunology, Department of Pediatrics, Louisiana State University Health Sciences Center, Head, Jeffrey Modell Center for Primary Immunodeficiencies, New Orleans, Louisiana

PANIDA SRIAROON, MD
Associate Professor, Division of Allergy and Immunology, Department of Pediatrics, University of South Florida, Saint Petersburg, Florida

TROY R. TORGERSON, MD, PhD
Seattle Children's Hospital; Associate Professor, Pediatrics, Immunology/Rheumatology, University of Washington School of Medicine; Director, Immunology Diagnostic Lab, Seattle Children's Research Institute, Seattle, Washington

LUKE A. WALL, MD
Assistant Professor, Section of Allergy Immunology, Department of Pediatrics, Louisiana State University Health Sciences Center, Jeffrey Modell Center for Primary Immunodeficiencies, New Orleans, Louisiana

CHRISTIAN A. WYSOCKI, MD, PhD
Division of Allergy and Immunology, Department of Internal Medicine, UT Southwestern Medical Center, Dallas, Texas

Contents

> The spectrum of primary immunodeficiency disorders (PIDs) is expanding. It includes typical disorders that primarily present with defective immunity as well as disorders that predominantly involve other systems and show few features of impaired immunity. The rapidly growing list of new immunodeficiency disorders and treatment modalities makes it imperative for providers to stay abreast of the latest and best management strategies. This article presents a brief overview of recent clinical advances in PIDs.

> Recurrent infections in children are a cause for concern. It is essential to distinguish simple recurrent infections caused by exposures in the day care or school settings from those caused by inherent deficiencies in the immune system or other systemic diseases. Multiple diagnostic tools are available for the evaluation of recurrent infections. The sites of infections and organisms responsible are important in guiding clinicians in the appropriate laboratory work-up and diagnosis of these patients. Once a diagnosis is made, proper treatment and management decisions can be made to treat the patients appropriately and ensure their lifelong health.

> Common variable immunodeficiency (CVID) refers to a grouping of antibody deficiencies that lack a more specific genetic or phenotypic classification. It is the immunodeficiency classification with the greatest number of constituents, likely because of the numerous ways in which antibody production can be impaired and the frequency in which antibody production becomes impaired in human beings. CVID comprises a heterogeneous group of rare diseases. Consequently, CVID presents a significant challenge for researchers and clinicians. Despite these difficulties, both our understanding of and ability to manage this grouping of complex immune diseases has advanced significantly over the past 60 years.

> Patients with specific antibody deficiency (SAD) have a deficient immunologic response to polysaccharide antigens. Such patients experience sinopulmonary infections with increased frequency, duration, or severity compared with the general population. SAD is definitively diagnosed by

immunologic challenge with a pure polysaccharide vaccine in patients 2 years old and older who have otherwise intact immunity, using the 23-valent pneumococcal polysaccharide vaccine as the current gold standard. Specific antibody deficiencies comprise multiple immunologic phenotypes. Treatment must be tailored based on the severity of symptoms. Most patients have a good prognosis. The deficiency may resolve over time, especially in children.

Severe combined immunodeficiency disorders represent pediatric emergencies due to absence of adaptive immune responses to infections. The conditions result from either intrinsic defects in T-cell development (ie, severe combined immunodeficiency disease [SCID]) or congenital athymia (eg, complete DiGeorge anomaly). Hematopoietic stem cell transplant provides the only clinically approved cure for SCID, although gene therapy research trials are showing significant promise. For greatest survival, patients should undergo transplant before 3.5 months of age and before the onset of infections. Newborn screening programs have yielded successful early identification and treatment of infants with SCID and congenital athymia in the United States.

Primary immunodeficiency disorders were among the first diseases in which hematopoietic stem cell transplant (HSCT) was attempted. Initial attempts at HSCT were discouraging and fraught with complications, but with increased knowledge and sophistication of HLA typing and donor matching, development of improved transplant conditioning regimens, and advances in prophylaxis and treatment of graft-versus-host disease, there has been a marked improvement in outcomes. This improvement has allowed an ever-growing number of different immunodeficiency and immune dysregulation disorders to be treated by HSCT. This article provides an overview of the approach to HSCT in these disorders.

Immunoglobulin replacement therapy has been standard treatment in patients with primary immunodeficiency diseases for the past 3 decades. The goal of therapy is to reduce serious bacterial infections in individuals with antibody function defects. Approximately one-third of patients receiving intravenous immunoglobulin treatment experience adverse reactions. Recent advances in manufacturing processes have resulted in products that are safer and better tolerated. Self-infusion by the subcutaneous route has become popular and resulted in better quality of life. This review summarizes the use of immunoglobulin therapy in primary immunodeficiency diseases including its properties, dosing, adverse effects, and different routes of administration.

The association of autoimmunity and primary immunodeficiency suggests the existence of mechanistic links between development of the various elements of the immune system and the maintenance of self-tolerance. In this review, various monogenic primary immunodeficiencies (PID) are systematically explored, with a specific focus on the impact of these genetic lesions on tolerance, correlating these defects in tolerance with clinical autoimmune and inflammatory syndromes seen in these PIDs. Common variable immunodeficiency (CVID) is explored, and areas are highlighted in which findings in monogenic PID are beginning to illuminate the mechanisms behind these conditions in CVID.

Pulmonary disease, ranging from infectious pneumonia, lung abscess, and empyema to structural lung diseases to malignancy, significantly increase morbidity and mortality in primary immune deficiency. Treatment with supplemental immunoglobulin (intravenous or subcutaneous) and antimicrobials is beneficial in reducing infections but is largely ineffective in preventing noninfectious complications, including interstitial lung disease, malignancy, and autoimmune disease. A low threshold for suspecting pulmonary complications is necessary for the early diagnosis of pulmonary involvement in primary immunodeficiency disorders, before irreversible damage is done, to improve patient outcomes.

Primary immune deficiencies (PIDs) are an uncommon heterogeneous group of diseases that result from fundamental defects in the proteins and cells that enable specific immune responses. Common allergic reactions (eczema, allergic rhinitis, asthma, and food allergies) are exaggerated immune responses that may be manifestations of an underlying PID. Early diagnosis and treatment has significant bearing on outcome. Immune suppression with systemic corticosteroids in these immune compromised individuals can lead to life threatening dissemination of infections.

IMMUNOLOGY AND ALLERGY CLINICS OF NORTH AMERICA

ISSUE OF RELATED INTEREST

Hematology/Oncology Clinics of North America, December 2014 (Vol. 28, Issue 6)
Bone Marrow Transplantation
Bipin N. Savani and Mohamad Mohty, *Editors*
http://www.hemonc.theclinics.com/

THE CLINICS ARE AVAILABLE ONLINE!
Access your subscription at:
www.theclinics.com

Preface

Primary Immunodeficiency Disorders

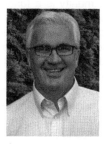

Anthony Montanaro, MD
Editor

We are very pleased to be presenting this issue on Primary Immunodeficiency Disorders (PIDD). PIDD is an essential clinical topic for Allergy/Immunology practitioners as well as primary care providers. Given the delay in diagnosis of over ten years in most patients, it is incumbent on us to have a better understanding of these disorders and to get the message of early diagnosis and treatment out to our colleagues. It has become very clear that early diagnosis and treatment of PIDD can reduce morbidity and mortality and improve all patients' quality of life. We believe that this issue of *Immunology and Allergy Clinics of North America* will add to our knowledge base and allow us to deliver higher-quality care to patients with PIDD.

We have been very fortunate that many leaders in the field of PIDD have graciously contributed to this issue. We feel that the topics we selected summarize the most important areas in the field. Drs Chitra Dinakar and Nikita Raje present a concise and useful overview of PIDD that will allow the reader to direct their interests to further presentations. Since many of the PIDD present in childhood, Dr Hernandez-Trujillo has presented a practical approach to the child with recurrent infection. We have asked Drs Gelfand and Abbott to focus on Common Variable Immunodeficiency due to its protean manifestations and because this field has been expanding so rapidly. Dr Sorensen and colleagues have presented an outstanding review on functional antibody deficiency, which has emerged as an important and treatable syndrome in patients who present with recurrent infection and normal screening tests for immunoglobulin levels.

Drs William Shearer and Ivan Chinn have been established leaders in the field of cellular immunodeficiency and have expertly presented an outstanding review on severe combined immunodeficiency. Their article outlines important aspects of diagnosis and management that are critical in saving the lives of these children. Dr Troy Torgerson and colleagues further detail the important emerging field of bone marrow transplantation (BMT) for SCID as well as other disorders. Their article outlines

Immunol Allergy Clin N Am 35 (2015) ix–x
http://dx.doi.org/10.1016/j.iac.2015.07.011
0889-8561/15/$ – see front matter © 2015 Published by Elsevier Inc.

immunology.theclinics.com

the emergence of BMT as a viable primary treatment modality for many of the PIDD. Further treatment options for humoral immunodeficiency in children and adults are presented by Drs Ballow and Sriaroon, who have spent their careers treating patients with PIDD.

The noninfectious manifestations of PIDD may be the most important aspect of their disease for many of our patients. In that regard, we have asked some of the authors to focus on those aspects. Since expression of autoimmunity is a fundamental abnormality in many of our patients, Drs Saifi and Wysocki present a comprehensive review of this topic. Many of our patients have both infectious and noninfectious manifestations of their PIDD as the most significant aspect of their disease. We have asked Dr Stephanie Nonas, who has provided excellent insight and advice in this area, to review this area. Finally, Drs Chan and Gelfand have reviewed the interesting area of how PIDD may masquerade as an allergic disease.

We hope that you enjoy reading this issue on PIDD. It is a comprehensive yet concise review of this important area of practice. It is meant to be a review, but all of the articles are well referenced and provide the reader opportunities to expand their search for further information if necessary. We have included information that is clinically relevant and important for specialists and primary care providers alike.

Anthony Montanaro, MD
Division of Allergy and Immunology
Oregon Health and Science University
3181 SW Sam Jackson Drive
Portland, OR 97202, USA

E-mail address:
montanar@ohsu.edu

Overview of Immunodeficiency Disorders

Nikita Raje, MD*, Chitra Dinakar, MD

KEYWORDS

- Immunodeficiency • Antibody deficiency • Autoimmunity • Immune defect
- Innate immune defect • Lymphoproliferation • Immune dysregulation

KEY POINTS

- Primary immunodeficiencies lead to various combinations of recurrent infections, autoimmunity, lymphoproliferation, granulomatous disease, atopy, and malignancy.
- Immunodeficiency caused by defects in more than 1 gene can lead to similar manifestations and a defect in the same gene can cause varied manifestations.
- High index of suspicion along with meticulous history and physical examination are a key to early diagnosis of primary immunodeficiency.
- Early primary immunodeficiency diagnosis can be achieved with improved access to validated immunologic laboratory tests.

INTRODUCTION

In the past, primary immunodeficiency disorders (PIDs) have been described as diseases caused by 1 or more defects of the immune system, leading to increased susceptibility to infections. It is now known that PIDs are a group of heterogeneous disorders with immune system abnormalities characterized by various combinations of recurrent infections, autoimmunity, lymphoproliferation, granulomatous process, atopy, and malignancy (**Fig. 1**). The overall clinical picture is dictated by the specific type of underlying immune defect. Based on the type of PID, the types of infections can vary. Although bacterial infections may be a key feature of B-cell defects, infections with diverse pathogens (eg, viruses, fungi, and bacteria) are a feature of combined T-cell and B-cell immunodeficiencies. Similarly, autoimmune manifestations can range from autoimmune

Disclosures: This work was supported by a CTSA grant from NCATS awarded to the University of Kansas Medical Center for Frontiers: The Heartland Institute for Clinical and Translational Research #UL1TR000001 (formerly #UL1RR033179). The contents are solely the responsibility of the authors and do not necessarily represent the official views of the NIH or NCATS.
Children's Mercy Hospital, University of Missouri-Kansas City, 2401 Gillham Road, Kansas City, MO 64108, USA
* Corresponding author.
E-mail address: nraje@cmh.edu

Immunol Allergy Clin N Am 35 (2015) 599–623
http://dx.doi.org/10.1016/j.iac.2015.07.001
0889-8561/15/$ – see front matter
immunology.theclinics.com

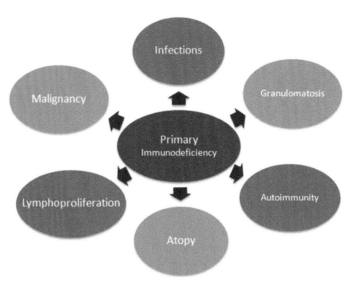

Fig. 1. Features of primary immunodeficiencies. (*Data from* Refs.[1,2,5–17,19–26])

cytopenias secondary to B-cell defects to systemic lupus erythematosus in complement disorders. Some PIDs (eg, X-linked lymphoproliferative disease) are characterized by lymphoproliferation, whereas others (such as those associated with chronic granulomatous disease) manifest with cutaneous, respiratory, or gastrointestinal tract granulomas caused by immune dysregulation. Although lymphomas and leukemias are the most common malignancies noted, other types of malignancies may also be seen. Atopic features such as asthma, atopic dermatitis, and food allergies can be observed in some patients with T-cell defects. Hence, the types of manifestations and involvement of other systems can provide a clue to the type of PID.

HISTORY

A few immune disorders, like ataxia telangiectasia (1926) and Wiskott-Aldrich syndrome (WAS) (1937), were discovered in the early part of the twentieth century. However, the landmark in the history of PIDs was the discovery of agammaglobulinemia by Colonel Ogden Bruton in 1952. In 1950, Eduard Glanzmann and Paul Riniker found that *Candida albicans* infections are associated with an absence of lymphocytes.[1] Two Swiss groups from Bern and Zurich (Hassig Cottier; R. Tobler and Walter Hitzig) discovered similar patients in 1958 and recognized the condition to be an immunodeficiency. The condition that was initially coined as Swiss-type agammaglobulinemia was renamed as severe combined immunodeficiency (SCID) by the World Health Organization (WHO) in 1970.[1] In 1954, Robert Good discovered a fatal granulomatous disease that is now known as chronic granulomatous disease (CGD).[1] Over the last 65 years, the field of PIDs has advanced greatly. With the advent of cutting-edge genetic technology, more than 240 PIDs have been discovered and the number continues to increase.[2]

EPIDEMIOLOGY

The prevalence of PID varies depending on the type of immunodeficiency. Although selective immunoglobulin (Ig) A deficiency is common (1 in 223 to 1 in 1000),[3] other immunodeficiencies, such as SCID, are rare (1 in 58,000).[4] Because immunodeficiencies are continually being discovered, the exact prevalence is unknown, although it is estimated to be low.

CLASSIFICATION

Immune deficiencies can be described as primary or secondary. Although primary immune deficiencies are caused by inherent dysfunction of the immune system and are chiefly genetic in cause, secondary immune deficiencies are consequent to other underlying causes (**Box 1**).

Various classifications for PIDs have been suggested. In 2014 the International Union of Immunodeficiency Society (IUIS) stratified PIDs into 9 categories based on the type of immune defect[2] (**Box 2**). Notably, some of the PIDs fit the criteria for more than 1 category in this schema. International consensus classification of PIDs recognizes the disorders of immune dysregulation and autoinflammation to be separate entities because their immune manifestations may be secondary to dysregulation or autoimmunity.[5]

Predominantly Antibody Deficiencies

Antibody deficiencies are typically characterized by a predisposition to infectious diseases. Infections are predominantly bacterial in origin but can be viral or protozoal as well. These deficiencies range from complete absence of antibody to varying degrees of functional antibody abnormalities (**Table 1**).

Combined Immunodeficiencies

SCID is associated with markedly reduced T cell levels and variable amounts of B cells. It is uniformly fatal if untreated. Typically, patients present early in life with failure to thrive, recurrent diarrhea, rashes, and serious bacterial, fungal, and viral infections. An assay developed to detect T-cell receptor excision circles (TRECs) has been used to screen newborns for SCID since 2009.[4] At present, 26 states in the United States use this technique, resulting into prompt recognition and successful treatment.

Other combined immunodeficiencies are associated with less severely affected T-cell and B-cell subsets. Some of them present with distinct associated features giving rise to a syndrome (see **Table 1**).

Phagocytic Defects

This category of PIDs includes disorders with either insufficient numbers of phagocytic cells or defective function. Patients with these conditions often have delayed wound healing and infectious granulomas with paucity of pus formation (see **Table 1**).

Complement Deficiencies

Complement defects

Complement defects include defects in classic pathway, alternative pathway, or lectin pathway.[6] Patients with classic pathway defects often have some concomitant features of autoimmunity in addition to immunodeficiency, whereas patients with the alternate and lectin pathway abnormalities commonly present with severe pyogenic infections (see **Table 1**).

Disorders of Innate Immunity

Innate immunodeficiencies include Toll-like receptor (TLR) defects and natural killer (NK) cell defects along with some other disorders with predisposition to viral/fungal infections as shown in **Tables 1**, **2**, and **3**.

Box 1
Causes of secondary immune deficiencies

1. Age
   a. Prematurity
   b. Infancy
   c. Old age
2. Medications
   a. Immunosuppressants
   b. Corticosteroids
3. Procedures
   a. Splenectomy
   b. Anesthesia use
   c. Post–stem cell transplant
4. Infections
   a. HIV infection, acquired immunodeficiency syndrome
   b. Cytomegalovirus
   c. Epstein-Barr virus
   d. Temporary during other infections
5. Metabolic
   a. Diabetes mellitus
   b. Uremia
6. Nutrition related
   a. Malnutrition
   b. Zinc deficiency
   c. Vitamin/other mineral deficiencies
7. Protein-losing conditions
   a. Nephrotic syndrome
   b. Protein-losing enteropathy
   c. Alcoholic cirrhosis
8. Hereditary conditions
   a. Chromosomal abnormalities
   b. Sickle cell disease
9. Miscellaneous
   a. Systemic lupus erythematosus
   b. Burns
   c. Malignancies
   d. Radiation therapy

Adapted from Stiehm RE, Ochs HD, Winkelstein JA. Immunodeficiency disorders: general considerations. In: Stiehm RE, Ochs HD, Winkelstein JA, eds. Immunologic disorders in infants and children. 5th edition. Philadelphia: Saunders; 2004.

> **Box 2**
> **Categories of PIDs as per IUIS 2014 classification**
>
> Predominantly antibody deficiencies
>
> T-cell immunodeficiencies or combined immunodeficiencies
>
> Syndromic immunodeficiencies
>
> Complement defects
>
> Phagocytic defects
>
> Defects of innate immunity
>
> Diseases of immune dysregulation
>
> Autoinflammatory disorders
>
> Phenocopies of PIDs
>
> *Data from* Al-Herz W, Bousfiha A, Casanova JL, et al. Primary immunodeficiency diseases: an update on the classification from the international union of immunological societies expert committee for primary immunodeficiency. Front Immunol 2014;5:162.

Nuclear factor kappa B pathway defect/anhidrotic ectodermal dysplasia

X-linked *NEMO* (Online Mendelian Inheritance in Man [OMIM] number 300248), autosomal dominant *IKBA* (OMIM# 612132) gain of function (GOF) mutation, and autosomal recessive *IKBKB* mutations can all cause ectodermal dysplasia, characterized by hypohidrosis, sparse hair, conical teeth, and early loss of teeth.[5] Hypogammaglobulinemia with impaired specific antibody production is noted in these defects. nuclear factor-kappa B essential modulator (NEMO) defect presents with *Streptococcus pneumoniae*, *Staphylococcus aureus*, *Pseudomonas aeruginosa*, *Haemophilus influenzae*, mycobacteria, and less frequently viral and fungal infections. NEMO defect may be marked by high IgM level in about 15% of patients. Patients with inhibitor of NF-kappa B alpha (IKBA) defects are prone to *Pneumocystis jirovecii* and mucocutaneous candidiasis.[5,7] inhibitor of NF-kappa B beta (IKBB) defect presents as SCID with the most common infections being *Listeria monocytogenes*, *Serratia marcescens*, *Escherichia coli*, mucocutaneous candidiasis, and parainfluenza.[5,8]

Toll-like receptor signaling pathway deficiency

Pyogenic infections Pyogenic infections are noted in interleukin-1 receptor associated kinase 4 (IRAK4), myeloid differentiation primary response gene 88 (MYD88), and heme-oxidized iron regulatory protein 2 ubiquitin ligase 1 (HOIL1) deficiencies.[7] *IRAK4* (OMIM# 607676) and *MyD88* (OMIM# 612260) present with infections caused by *S pneumoniae*, *S aureus*, and *P aeruginosa* but show normal resistance to most other bacteria, viruses, fungi, and parasites. The infections are marked by the absence of fever and normal C-reactive protein levels, although pus formation has been noted.[7]

Herpes simplex encephalitis Defects in TLR3 pathway can present with herpes simplex encephalitis (HSE). Some defects, namely *TLR3* (OMIM# 613002), *UNC93B1* (OMIM# 610551), *TRAF3* (OMIM# 614849), *TRIF* (OMIM# 614850), and *TBK1*[5,9] predispose patients to recurrent HSE.

Natural killer cell deficiency

Natural killer (NK) cell deficiency[10] can be classified as classic NK-cell deficiency (CNKD) with absence of NK cells or functional NK-cell deficiency (FNKD) with a normal number of NK cells but impaired function; secondary NK-cell deficiency must be ruled

Table 1
Subclassification of some PIDs

Type of PID	Clinical Features	Infections	Genetic Mutations (Other Names) (OMIM Numbers)
Antibody Deficiencies			
Severely reduced serum immunoglobulin levels with profoundly decreased or absent B cells (agammaglobulinemia)[2,27,28]	• Defect in early development of B cells in the bone marrow • Complete or near-total absence of B cells in peripheral blood • Lack of peripheral lymphoid tissue like lymph nodes and tonsils • Almost all of them (90%) present by preschool age, with more than half presenting in infancy following the depletion of maternal immuno globulins, and a few in adulthood	• Recurrent otitis media, pneumonia, and sinusitis • Chronic enteroviral meningoencephalitis and neutropenia have been reported in XLA	• *BTK* 85% (Bruton or XLA) (300300) • Autosomal recessive Agam: deficiency of mu heavy chain (147020), *λ5* (146770), *CD79α* (*Igα*) (112205) and *CD79β* (*Igβ*) (147245), *BLNK* (604615), *PIK3R1* (171833), and *TCF3* (147141) • Other causes: myelodysplasia with hypogammaglobulinemia (monosomy 7, trisomy 8, or dyskeratosis congenita), and thymoma with immunodeficiency with unknown genetic defect
Severely reduced serum immunoglobulin isotypes (at least 2) with normal or low numbers of B cells: commonly classified as CVID[2,29]	• Present after 2 y of age with IgG 2 SD less than normal for age, low IgA and/or IgM levels, and defective specific or functional antibodies • Other causes of hypogammaglobulinemia should be ruled out • Heterogeneous manifestations like autoimmunity, granulomatous disease, gastrointestinal disease, lymphoid hyperplasia, lymphoma, and other malignancies	• Recurrent infections: commonly sinopulmonary • Protozoal infections like *Giardia*	• *ICOS* (604558) • *CD19* (107265) • *CD81* (186845) • *CD20* (112210) • *CD21* (614699) • *TACI* (604907) • *LRBA* (606453), *BAFF-R* (606269), *TWEAK* (602695), *NFKB2* (615577), and *CXCR4* (WHIM syndrome) (193670) • Most patients do not have a causative gene identified • Once the causative gene is identified, it is appropriate to use the genetic name rather than CVID

Severe reduction in IgG and IgA, with normal or increased IgM level, and normal number of B cells (commonly termed as hyper-IgM syndrome)	• AID/UNG[30]: patients present with lymphoid hyperplasia, and increased risk for autoimmunity	Bacterial infections	AID (605257) and UNG (191525) defects mainly affect class switch recombination and somatic hypermutation
	• CD40/CD40L[30,31] lack secondary germinal centers in lymph nodes. They also have increased susceptibility to sclerosing cholangitis and hepatocellular carcinomas	Opportunistic infections (Cryptosporidium parvum, Histoplasma, Bartonella, Candida, and Cryptococcus sp)	CD40 (109535), CD40L (300386) affect T and B lymphocyte interaction and resulting signaling
		—	Other causes of high IgM levels: NEMO defect (300248) PI3K p110delta deficiency, Other diseases: PMS2, AT and NBS
Isotype or light chain deficiencies with generally normal number of B cells	• SIgAD can occur in isolation, with IgG subclass, or specific antibody deficiency	Most patients are asymptomatic and diagnosed incidentally, such as while testing for celiac disease but SIgAD can present with recurrent sinopulmonary infections	The cause is not known but associated TACI mutations have been found
	• SIgAD can be associated with autoimmunity, atopic diseases, and rarely lymphoid and gastrointestinal malignancies[3]		
	• May evolve into CVID later in life		
	• Isolated IgG subclass deficiency is mostly asymptomatic unless associated with other immune defects like specific antibody deficiency	—	—
	• PI3K p110delta deficiency[32] can be associated with lymphomas	CMV, EBV	• PIK3CD, PI3K-δ Other PIDs in this category include immunoglobulin heavy chain, kappa constant deficiency, PIK3CD, PRKCD mutations

(continued on next page)

Table 1
(continued)

Type of PID	Clinical Features	Infections	Genetic Mutations (Other Names) (OMIM Numbers)
Specific antibody deficiencies with normal number of B cells	• Inability to produce sufficient antibodies to specific microbes, commonly those with protective polysaccharide capsules such as *Pneumococcus* and *Haemophilus influenzae*	Recurrent sinopulmonary infections or as per the specific antibody that is defective	—
THI with normal number of B cells	• Decreased IgG (2 SD lower than normal level for age), low IgA and/or IgM level once the transplacentally transferred maternal IgG level wanes • Typically resolves during toddlerhood but can persist till 5 y of age,[27] and, rarely, evolve into lasting PID	Although THI can be asymptomatic, toddlers can have recurrent sinopulmonary infections or, less commonly, severe invasive infections, triggering evaluation	—
Combined Immunodeficiencies			
Low CD8 subset	• Severe ZAP70[33] deficiency can present with features of SCID • Hypomorphic mutations cause low CD8 counts and increased IgE • CD8 deficiency[34] and those with MHC class I deficiency can present during childhood or adulthood • Vasculitis and pyoderma gangrenosum noted in MHC class I deficiency • Bronchiectasis and skin granulomas are noted[35]	Recurrent bacterial (sinopulmonary), fungal, and viral infections Chronic sinusitis and respiratory infections	*ZAP70* (269840), *CD8* (186910), *TAP1, TAP2, TAPBP* (604571)

Low CD4 T-cell subset	MHC class II deficiency,[36] also known as bare lymphocyte syndrome, presents with protracted diarrhea, failure to thrive, and autoimmunity	Recurrent bacterial, fungal, viral, protozoal infections	CIITA, RFX5, RFXAP, RFXANK (209920)
	• MAGT1 deficiency[37] can present with chronic EBV infection and related malignancies • Also called XMEN	Chronic EBV infection	MAGT1 (300715)
	LCK[38] and LRBA[39] deficiency can present with autoimmunity and inflammatory manifestations	Recurrent infections	LCK (153390) and LRBA (606453)
	UNC119 deficiency[40] can present with bronchiectasis	Recurrent infections (viral, fungal, and bacterial)	UNC119 (604011)
Low CD27+ B-cell level	CD27 deficiency[41] is associated with hypogammaglobulinemia.	Persistent EBV viremia	CD27 (615122)
Progressive decrease in T-cell numbers, with normal B-cell numbers, and normal or decreased serum immunoglobulin levels	• ITK deficiency[42] can present with lymphadenopathy, hepatosplenomegaly, cytopenias, EBV-associated malignancies, and other viral and fungal infections • Neurologic impairment and autoimmune hemolytic anemia are noted in PNP deficiency[2]	—	ITK (613011), PNP (164050)
Combined Immunodeficiencies with Associated Syndromic Features			
Congenital thrombocytopenia and eczema	• Seen in WAS[43] or WASP interacting protein (WIP) deficiency[44] • Can present with autoimmunity and malignancy	—	—

(continued on next page)

Table 1
(continued)

Type of PID	Clinical Features	Infections	Genetic Mutations (Other Names) (OMIM Numbers)
DNA repair defects[45]	• AT presents with progressive neurologic impairment, later onset of telangiectasia • Patients with AT can develop malignancies like leukemia and lymphoma • Immune defects noted are low IgG and IgA with high IgM levels • Alpha fetoprotein level is increased	—	AT (604391), NBS (251260), and Bloom syndrome (210900)
—	• Patients with NBS present with growth retardation and microcephaly, and have increased risk of malignancy like lymphoma • Alpha fetoprotein level is normal in NBS	—	—
Thymic defects	• Chromosome 22q11.2 deletion syndrome[25,26] (congenital heart defect, hypocalcemia, cleft lip/palate, behavioral problems) • Immune system can range from normal, or partial combined deficiency causing recurrent sinopulmonary infections to profound T-cell deficiency leading to SCID-like features • CHARGE syndrome[25] • Varying degrees of immune defects ranging from normal immune system to absence of T cells	—	Chromosome 22q11.2 deletion (188400) *CHD7* (608892), *SEMA3E* (214800)

Osseous dysplasias[46]	• Cartilage-hair hypoplasia: short-limbed short stature, joint laxity, metaphyseal chondrodysplasia, hair hypoplasia, neuronal dysplasia of intestine, and increased risk of malignancy • Both cellular and humoral immune defects are noted	—	*RMRP* (250250)
	• Schimke syndrome presents with dysmorphic facies, thin hair, spondyloepiphyseal dysplasia, short spine, renal failure, and hyperpigmented macules along with cellular immune defects	Opportunistic infections	*SMARCAL1* (242900)
Hyper-IgE syndromes[47]	• STAT3 deficiency eczema, pneumatoceles, coarse facies, skeletal anomalies like scoliosis	Recurrent skin abscesses	*STAT3* (147060), *Tyk2* (611521), *DOCK8* (243700), *PGM3* (172100)
—	• DOCK8 lacks the skeletal features but is more often associated with allergies • Impaired T-cell (CD8) and NK-cell function, low NK-cell count, and low CD27+ memory B cells	Viral infections like HPV, Varicella zoster, molluscum contagiosum, HSV	Other disorders, like WAS and Omenn syndrome, and can have high IgE levels
	• Tyk2 deficiency can present with severe eczema	*Staphylococcus* infections, intracellular infections like mycobacteria, *Salmonella*, fungi, and viruses	—
	• PGM3 deficiency can present with impaired neurocognition, autoimmunity, and severe eczema	—	—

(continued on next page)

Table 1
(continued)

Type of PID	Clinical Features	Infections	Genetic Mutations (Other Names) (OMIM Numbers)
Phagocytic Defects			
Motility defects	• Leukocyte adhesion deficiency present with poor wound healing, delayed separation of umbilical cord, periodontitis, neutrophilia, and leukocytosis ○ LAD1 presents with delayed separation of umbilical cord, poor wound healing with paucity of pus in early infancy and is marked by lack of CD18 on flow cytometry[48] ○ LAD2 is characterized by psychomotor and growth retardation but decreasing infections with age. It is marked by the presence of Bombay blood group and lack of fucosylated glycoprotein moieties like sialyl Lewis X[48] ○ LAD3 features bleeding tendency and sometimes osteopetrosis in early infancy[5,48]	—	*ITGB2* (116920), *FUCT1* (266265), *KINDLIN3* (612840) Other motility defect: *RAC2* (602049)
Respiratory burst defects: CGD[5]	• Defective NADPH oxidase system • Associated with granulomatous disease of gastrointestinal, respiratory, or urinary tracts	Catalase-positive organisms like *Staphylococcus aureus, Nocardia, Pseudomonas, Serratia* sp, *Burkholderia cepacia* Fungi like *Candida* and *Aspergillus*	*CYBB* (306400), *CYBA* (233690), *NCF1* (233700), *NCF2* (233710), and *NCF4* (601488)

Mendelian susceptibility to mycobacterial disease[5]	Defects in IL12/IFN gamma pathway lead to susceptibility to specific organisms	Infection by *Salmonella* spp, mycobacteria, and *Cryptococcus neoformans*	*IL12RB1* (209950), *IL12B* (161561), *IFNGR1* (209950), *IFNGR2* (147569), *STAT1* (600555), *CYBB* (306400), *IRF8* (601565), *ISG15* (147571)
GATA2 deficiency[49,50]	• Low B-cell, NK-cell, and monocyte counts • CD4 and neutrophil counts can be low but are less remarkable • Lymph edema, pulmonary alveolar proteinosis, warts, skin malignancies, sensorineural hearing loss, miscarriage, hypothyroidism, myelodysplasia, and leukemias are other features	Severe viral infections, mycobacterial infections, fungal infections	*GATA2* (137295)
Complement Defects[2,5,6]			
Early complement defects	• C1q, C1r, C1s, C4, C2 deficiency present with systemic lupus erythematosus • C3, factor I, H deficiency, CD46 deficiency can present with infections, glomerulonephritis, and atypical hemolytic-uremic syndrome	Infections with encapsulated organisms	120550, 601269, 120575, 216950, 120580, 120810, 120820, 217000, 120700, 610984, 609814, 120920
Late complement and alternative pathway deficiency-like	C5, C6, C7, C8 (C8A, C8G, C8B), C9 (mild), factor D, properdin deficiency	Present with infections caused by neisserial species	120900, 217050, 217070, 120950, 120960, 613825, 134350, 312060
Other complement defects	Inflammatory lung disease and autoimmunity Ficolin 3 can present with necrotizing enterocolitis	• MASP2 deficiency: respiratory and pyogenic infections • Ficolin 3 deficiency can present with respiratory infections and abscesses	605102, 604973

Abbreviations: AID, activation-induced cytidine deaminase; AT, ataxia telangiectasia; CHARGE, coloboma, heart defect, atresia choanae, retarded growth and development, genital hypoplasia, ear anomalies/deafness; CMV, cytomegalovirus; CVID, common variable immunodeficiency; EBV, Epstein-Barr virus; HSV, herpes simplex virus; IFN, interferon; IL, interleukin; ITK, interleukin-2–inducible T-cell kinase; LAD, leukocyte adhesion defect; LRBA, lipopolysaccharide-responsive and beigelike anchor protein; MAGT1, magnesium transporter 1; MASP, mannose associated serine protease; MHC, major histocompatibility complex; NBS, Nijmegen breakage syndrome; OMIM, Online Mendelian Inheritance in Man; PNP, purine nucleotide phosphorylase; SD, standard deviations; SIgAD, selective IgA deficiency; STAT, signal transducer and activator of transcription; THI, transient hypogammaglobulinemia of infancy; UNG, uracil DNA glycosylase; WASP, wiskott aldrich syndrome protein; WHIM, warts hypogammaglobulinemia, infections, myelokathexis; XLA, X-linked agammaglobulinemia; XMEN, X-linked EBV-associated neoplasia.

Data from Refs.[2,3,5,6,25–49]

Table 2
Typical infections in PIDs

Infection/Infective Agent	Associated Primary Immunodeficiency
Recurrent EBV	XLP1, XIAP, CD27, ITK, MAGT1, Coronin1-A def, PI3K-delta, PRKCD
HSV encephalitis	TLR3 signaling pathway defects
Neisseria meningitidis	Terminal complement defects
Serratia marcescens, B cepacia, S aureus, Listeria monocytogenes, Granulibacter bethesdensis, Chromobacterium violaceum, Francisella philomiragia, Mycobacteria, Nocardia, Aspergillus, C albicans, Paecilomyces spp	CGD
Enteroviral encephalitis	X-linked agammaglobulinemia
Mycobacteria	CGD, NEMO/NFKB1 pathway defects, IL12 pathway defects, Tyk2, GATA2, IRF8, macrophage gp91 phox, ISG15 deficiencies
HSV, EBV, cytomegalovirus, Varicella	CNKD, FNKD, DOCK8 deficiency
C neoformans	Anti–GM-CSF Abs, IFN gamma pathway defects
Cryptosporidium parvum	Hyper-IgM syndrome, IL21-R defect
S aureus	Anti-IL6 Abs, DOCK8 deficiency
Chronic mucocutaneous candidiasis	IL17 signaling pathway defects, STAT1, VODI, IRF8, APECED, Act1 deficiency
Invasive candidiasis or other fungal disease	CARD9
Salmonella sp	IL12 pathway defects, IFN gamma pathway defects, STAT1, Tyk2, IRF8, ISG15 deficiencies
HPV	DOCK8, EVER1, EVER2, GATA2, WHIM, RHOH, STK4 deficiencies
Trypanosomiasis	APOL1
HSV	STAT1, CNKD, FNKD
Pneumocystis jirovecii	SCID, hyper-IgM, VODI, CARD11, IL21-R
Histoplasma	GATA2 deficiency
Molluscum contagiosum	RHOH deficiency

Abbreviations: anti–GM-CSF Abs, anti–granulocyte macrophage colony–stimulating factor antibodies; APECED, autoimmune polyendocrinopathy candidiasis ectodermal dystrophy; CARD, caspase recruitment domain-containing protein; CNKD, classic NK-cell deficiency; DOCK8, dedicator of cytokinesis; EVER, epidermodysplasia verruciformis gene; FNKD, functional NK-cell deficiency; GATA2, GATA binding protein-2; gp91 phox, glycoprotein 91 phagocytic oxidase; IL21-R, IL21 receptor; IRF8, interferon regulatory factor 8; ISG15, interferon stimulated gene 15; NEMO, NF-kappa B essential modulator; NFKB1, NF-kappa B1; PI3K-delta, phosphoinositide 3-kinase; PRKCD, protein kinase C delta; RHOH, ras homolog gene family member H; STK4, serine/threonine protein kinase 4; TLR3, toll-like receptor 3; Tyk2, tyrosine kinase 2; VODI, venoocclusive disease with immunodeficiency; XIAP, X-linked inhibitor of apoptosis; XLP1, X-linked lymphoproliferative disease 1.

out. Patients with CKND (*GATA2*; OMIM# 137295) and *MCM4* (OMIM# 609981) can present with herpes simplex virus (HSV), Epstein-Barr virus (EBV), cytomegalovirus (CMV), varicella-zoster virus (VZV), human papilloma virus (HPV), and less commonly fungal infections. They have increased risk of malignancies. FNKD (*FCGR3A*; OMIM# 146740) has been associated most commonly with HSV infections and rarely with VZV, EBV, and recurrent respiratory viral infections.

Table 3
Typical features of some primary immunodeficiencies

Clinical Feature	Associated Primary Immunodeficiency
Ectodermal dysplasia	NEMO/NFKB1 defect, IKBA, ORAI-1, STIM-1 deficiencies, Comel-Netherton syndrome
Alopecia	RAG1/2 (Omenn), FOXN1 defects
Myopathy	ORAI-1, STIM-1 deficiencies, Barth syndrome
Hypocalcemia	Chromosome 22q11.2 deletion
Neurologic impairment	PNP deficiency, Chédiak-Higashi, Kostmann syndrome
Thrombocytopenia	CD40LG, CD40, IKAROS defects
Neutropenia	Hermansky-Pudlak, TWEAK, CD40, CD40L defects, WAS, XLA
Dwarfism	STAT5b, MCM4 deficiencies, FILS syndrome, cartilage-hair hypoplasia, Shwachman-Diamond syndrome, Bloom syndrome, Schimke syndrome
Multiple intestinal atresia	TTC7A defect
Deafness/hearing impairment	Reticular dysgenesis, ADA, GATA2 deficiencies
Conjunctivitis/uveitis	Periodic fevers
Lymphoid hypertrophy	UNG, AID deficiencies
Eczema	WAS, DOCK8, STAT3, ITCH, Tyk2, STAT5b deficiencies
Food allergies	DOCK8 deficiency
Vasculitis	C7, C2 deficiency, MHC1 deficiency
Cold urticaria	NLRP3 defects, PLCG2 deficiency
PAP	GATA2, CSF2RA deficiencies, autoabs to GM-CSF
IBD/enteropathy	IL10, CGD, IPEX, CVID, STXBP2/MUNC 18-2 (FHL), XLP2, NOD2, LRBA deficiencies
Endocrinopathy	APECED, IPEX, chromosome 22q11.2 deletion
Lung disease	LRBA, ITCH deficiencies
Pneumatoceles	STAT3 deficiencies
Periodontitis	LAD, localized juvenile periodontitis, hyper-IgM syndrome
Lymph edema	GATA2 deficiency
Adrenal insufficiency	MCM4 deficiency
Cleft lip/palate	Chromosome 22q11.2 deletion, MASP1, 3MC syndrome
Kaposi sarcoma	OX40 deficiency
Osteomyelitis	*IL-1RN* (deficiency of IL1 receptor antagonist), *LPIN2* (chronic recurrent multifocal osteomyelitis and congenital dyserythropoietic anemia or Majeed syndrome)
Psoriasis	DITRA (*IL36RN*), CAMPS (*CARD14*)
Panniculitis	CANDLE (*PSMB8*)

Abbreviations: 3MC, Carnevale, Mingarelli, Malpuech, and Michels syndrome; ADA, adenosine deaminase; AID, activation-induced cytidine deaminase; autoabs to GM-CSF, autoantibodies to granulocyte macrophage colony–stimulating factor; C, complement; CAMPS, CARD14 mediated psoriasis; CANDLE, chronic atypical neutrophilic dermatitis with lipodystrophy; CARD, caspase recruitment domain; CD40LG, CD40 ligand; CNKD, classic NK-cell deficiency; CSF2RA, colony stimulating factor 2 receptor alpha; DITRA, deficiency of IL36 receptor antagonist; DO8, dedicator of cytokinesis; FHL, familial hemophagocytic lymphohistiocytosis; FILS, facial dysmorphism, immunodeficiency, livedo, and short stature; FOXN1, forkhead box protein N1; IBD, inflammatory bowel disease; IPEX, immunodeficiency polyendocrinopathy enteropathy X-linked; LRBA, lipopolysaccharide responsive beige-like anchor protein; MASP, mannose binding lectin associated serine protease; MCM4, minichromosome maintenance deficient 4 homolog; NFKB1-NF-kappa B1; NLRP3, Nod-like receptor PYD family; NOD2, nucleotide-binding oligomerization domain receptor; PAP, pulmonary alveolar proteinosis; PLCG, phospholipase gamma; RAG1, recombination activating gene; STAT, signal transducer and activator of transcription; STIM-1, stromal interaction molecule 1; TTC7A, tetratricopeptide repeat domain-7A; TWEAK, TNF-like weak inducer of apoptosis; UNG, uracil-DNA glycosylase; WAS, Wiskott-Aldrich syndrome; XLP, X-linked lymphoproliferative syndrome.

DISORDERS OF IMMUNE DYSREGULATION

These disorders are associated with autoimmune manifestations and lymphoproliferation. Cytokine/interleukin (IL) pathway defects involve mutations that can result in gain or loss of function.

Familial Hemophagocytic Lymphohistiocytosis

Familial hemophagocytic lymphohistiocytosis (FHL)[11] is a disease of defective cytotoxic cells and lysosomes leading to excessive cytokine release, and T cell–related and macrophage-related inflammation. It typically presents with fever, cytopenias, and hepatosplenomegaly. It is distinguished by the presence of hemophagocytosis, hypofibrinogenemia, hypertriglyceridemia, increased ferritin and soluble IL2 (CD25) levels, abnormal liver functions, and decreased NK-cell activity. FHL without hypopigmentation is caused by defects in cytotoxic granule priming and fusion. The genetic mutations identified to date include *PRF1* (OMIM# 603553), *UNC13D* (OMIM# 608898), *STX11* (OMIM# 603552), and *STXBP2* (OMIM# 613101). FHL with hypopigmentation results in partial oculocutaneous albinism and immune defects; examples of such conditions are Chédiak-Higashi (*LYST*; OMIM# 214500), Griscelli type 2 (*RAB27A*; OMIM# 607624), and Hermansky-Pudlak type 2 (*AP3B1*; OMIM# 608233) syndromes. Defective secretory lysosomes in various cells cause features such as bleeding, neutropenia, and immunodeficiency.

Immunodeficiency; Polyendocrinopathy, Enteropathy, X Linked; and Polyendocrinopathy, Enteropathy, X Linked–like Disorders

Immunodeficiency, polyendocrinopathy, enteropathy, X-linked (IPEX) and IPEX-like disorders most commonly present with autoimmunity/cytopenias, diabetes mellitus, enteropathy, eczema, and bacterial infections. Although IPEX is caused by defective regulatory T cells because of mutations in *FOXP3* (OMIM# 304790), mutations in CD25 deficiency (*IL2RA*; OMIM# 606367), *STAT5B* (OMIM# 245590), *STAT1* (MIM# 614162), and *LRBA* (OMIM# 606453)[12,13] cause IPEX-like syndromes.

Lymphoproliferative Disorders Associated with Epstein-Barr Virus (EBV)

Lymphoproliferative disorders associated with EBV X-linked lymphoproliferative syndrome 1 (XLP1) (*SH2D1A* OMIM# 308240), XLP2 (*BIRC4* or *XIAP*; OMIM# 300635), *ITK* (OMIM# 613011), and *CD27* (OMIM# 615122) deficiency can present with EBV-induced lymphoproliferation. These conditions predispose to the development of lymphomas, except in patients with XLP2 deficiency, who are more likely to develop colitis. Patients with XLP1, XLP2, or CD27 defects can develop hemophagocytic lymphohistiocytosis (HLH).[14]

Autoimmunity Without Lymphoproliferation

Autoimmunity without lymphoproliferation is noted in autoimmune polyendocrinopathy candidiasis ectodermal dystrophy (APECED) (OMIM# 240300) and Itchy E3 ubiquitin protein ligase (ITCH) (OMIM# 613385) syndromes. APECED is caused by mutation in *AIRE*.[2] ITCH defect can cause hepatosplenomegaly, dysmorphism, failure to thrive, developmental delay. Lungs, liver, and gastrointestinal tract can be infiltrated by inflammatory cells.[15]

Autoimmune Lymphoproliferative Syndrome

Autoimmune lymphoproliferative syndrome (ALPS) is a disorder with lymphadenopathy and splenomegaly of at least 6 months' duration, cytopenias, and predisposition to lymphomas. It is marked by the presence of double-negative T lymphocytes (TCRαβ CD4-CD8- B220+ cells).[16] Defects in *FAS* (OMIM# 601859), *FASLG* (OMIM# 134638), and caspase 10 (OMIM# 603909) can cause ALPS. Caspase 8 (OMIM# 607271), *FADD* deficiency (OMIM# 613759), *CARD 11* GOF (OMIM# 606445), *PRKCD* (OMIM# 615559) defects display overlapping features. Recurrent infections are seen in caspase 8 deficiency.[16]

AUTOINFLAMMATORY DISORDERS
Periodic Fever Syndrome

These disorders are characterized by periodic fevers.[17] Depending on the causative genes, other manifestations include arthritis, abdominal pain, and urticarial or other rash. Cryopyrin-associated periodic fevers are caused by mutations in *NALP3* and are associated with conjunctivitis and amyloidosis and various syndromes (eg, Muckle-Wells syndrome [OMIM# 191900], familial cold autoinflammatory syndrome [OMIM# 120100], neonatal-onset multisystem inflammatory disease [OMIM# 607115]). Monogenic causes of periodic fevers caused by mutations in *MEFV* (OMIM# 249100; familial Mediterranean fever), *MVK* (OMIM# 260920; hyper-IgD), and TRAPS (*TNFRSF1*; OMIM# 142680) occur in specific ethnicities. Pyogenic infections, fever, aphthous ulcers, pharyngitis, and adenopathy is a periodic fever syndrome with unknown gene defect.

Inflammatory bowel disease, chronic osteomyelitis, psoriasis, panniculitis, and pyoderma gangrenosum can be manifestations of various autoinflammatory disorders.[2]

PHENOCOPIES OF PRIMARY IMMUNODEFICIENCY DISORDERS

These disorders behave and present like primary PIDs, but they are acquired secondary to occurrence of autoantibodies or somatic mutations.[2]

- Somatic mutations: ALPS-sFAS, RAS-associated autoimmune leukoproliferative disease (*KRAS* or *NRAS*).
- Autoantibodies: chronic mucocutaneous candidiasis (IL17, IL22), adult-onset immunodeficiency with mycobacterial and salmonella infections (interferon gamma), recurrent skin infections (IL6), pulmonary alveolar proteinosis (granulocyte macrophage colony–stimulating factor [GM-CSF]), and acquired angioedema (C1 inhibitor).

DIAGNOSIS

The diagnosis of PIDs is challenging for multiple reasons:

- Because PIDs are rare, a high index of suspicion is needed
- Individuals with the same PID can have different manifestations, and most PIDs lack pathognomonic characteristics
- Individuals with a defect in the same gene can have different presentations
- Screening tests are nonspecific
- Normal results of the screening test do not rule out PID
- Some of the diagnostic laboratory tests use specialized techniques that are not available in commercial laboratories

HISTORY AND PHYSICAL EXAMINATION

A meticulous history and a comprehensive physical examination are critical to diagnose PIDs. Clues to the correct diagnosis may include history of recurrent infections, presence of affected family members, physical findings related to growth and development, and presence or absence of peripheral lymphatic tissue. The 10 warning signs published by the Jeffrey Modell Foundation help to alert providers, ensuring that screening is initiated in situations in which these criteria are met.

Causes of secondary PIDs, such as medications, human immunodeficiency virus, malnutrition, and protein-losing conditions, should be ruled out. Other conditions predisposing to recurrent infections should be considered in the differential diagnosis. For instance, recurrent sinopulmonary infections can be a feature of cystic fibrosis, primary ciliary dyskinesia, bronchiectasis, or environmental allergies. Similarly recurrent skin infections can be secondary to atopic dermatitis.

Table 2 provides a list of infectious agents and associated PIDs. **Table 3** provides a list of clinical features and associated PIDs. These lists may serve as guides but are not exhaustive.

LABORATORY INVESTIGATIONS

The laboratory evaluation of patients with suspected PIDs is typically 2 or 3 tiered, starting with screening tests and followed by definitive diagnostic and molecular tests.[18] Some of the useful but often forgotten tests include peripheral blood smear, erythrocyte sedimentation rate, and C-reactive protein. Over the last 5 years, newborn screening for TRECs has changed the paradigm of screening evaluation.

Screening Tests

These tests are listed in **Fig. 2**A. Test results can be affected by various external factors, like age or specimen handling. For example, isohemagglutinin testing cannot be reliably performed until 6 months of age, lymphocyte proliferation assays to antigen stimulation may be impaired before the age of 1 year, and response to polysaccharide antigen is suboptimal until after 24 months of age. Hence, test results should always be compared with age-appropriate reference values. Specimen handling can affect some of the laboratory tests. For instance, a low serum complement level can be a result of specimen handling issues and delay in running the assay.

Second-tier Tests

These tests are performed based on clinical features and results of the screening tests (**Fig. 2**B). Particular attention should be paid to the laboratory techniques used because the results and normal ranges can vary depending on the technique. Some of these tests are performed in research laboratories and have limited availability in clinical laboratories. For example, although the basic T-cell, B-cell, and NK-cell markers by flow cytometry are available in most laboratories, the tests to evaluate lymphocyte signaling have limited availability. This limited availability also limits the experience and expertise in the interpretation of these tests to limited academic centers.

Definitive molecular diagnosis is pursued more often now that next-generation sequencing has made it possible to pinpoint the molecular cause. The various methods of genetic testing are shown in **Fig. 2**C.

TREATMENT
Definitive Treatment

The type of treatment offered depends on the type of immunodeficiency (**Fig. 3**).

For antibody deficiencies, the options range from (1) monitoring (asymptomatic selective IgA deficiency [SIgAD]), to (2) prophylactic antibiotics (symptomatic SIgAD), to (3) immunoglobulin replacement therapy (agammaglobulinemia, common variable

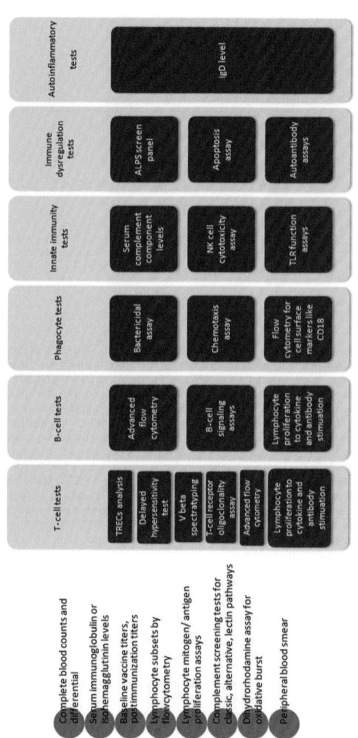

Fig. 2. Diagnostic tests in evaluation of primary immunodeficiencies. (*A*) Basic immunology work-up. (*B*) Advanced immunology work-up based on clinical and laboratory clues. (*C*) Molecular testing. ALPS, autoimmune lymphoproliferative syndrome; NK, natural killer; TLR, toll-like receptor; TRECs, T-cell receptor excision circles. (*Data from* Locke BA, Dasu T, Verbsky JW. Laboratory diagnosis of primary immunodeficiencies. Clin Rev Allergy Immunol 2014;46(2):154–68.)

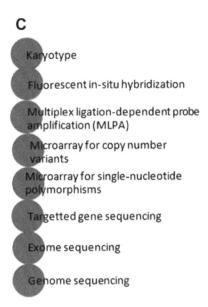

C

Karyotype

Fluorescent in-situ hybridization

Multiplex ligation-dependent probe amplification (MLPA)

Microarray for copy number variants

Microarray for single-nucleotide polymorphisms

Targetted gene sequencing

Exome sequencing

Genome sequencing

Fig. 2. (*continued*).

immunodeficiency [CVID], and specific antibody deficiencies). The dose of immuno-globulin replacement should be individualized based on clinical response.[19] Immuno-suppressants (eg, hydroxychloroquine, infliximab, and a combination of azathioprine and rituximab) are used for treatment of granulomatous lymphocytic interstitial lung disease associated with CVID.[20] High mortality was observed in the clinical trials of patients with CVID who were treated with hematopoietic stem cell transplantation (HSCT); however, benefit was noted in the surviving patients, suggesting a need for further studies.[21]

For SCID, the definitive treatment options include enzyme replacement (eg, polyeth-ylene glycol adenosine deaminase [ADA]), gene therapy, and HSCT. Gene therapy with retroviral vectors was previously attempted but was reported to increase the risk for development of leukemia and myelodysplasia.[22] Recent studies have shown some promise for gene therapy using lentivirus vectors.[22] HSCT outcomes depend on several factors, like the age at the time of HSCT, active infections, type of donor (matched/mismatched, related/unrelated, bone marrow/cord blood), and conditioning regimen.[23]

Phagocytic defects are managed with prophylactic antimicrobials and interferon gamma infusions. Some disorders with neutropenia can be treated with granulocyte colony–stimulating factor (G-CSF).

Some well-defined syndromes, such as WAS, hyper-IgM syndrome caused by CD40 and CD40L defects, DOCK8 defect, IPEX, HLH, XLP, and CGD, can also be treated with HSCT.[24] Gene therapy has been attempted for X-linked SCID, ADA defi-ciency, WAS, and CGD.[22]

Chromosome 22q11.2 deletion syndrome (OMIM# 188400) and CHARGE (colo-boma, heart defect, atresia choanae, retarded growth and development, genital hypo-plasia, ear anomalies/deafness) syndrome (*CHD7* [OMIM# 608892], *SEMA3E* [OMIM# 214800]) with profound T-cell immunodeficiency have been treated with thymic trans-plantation in a clinical trial.[25,26]

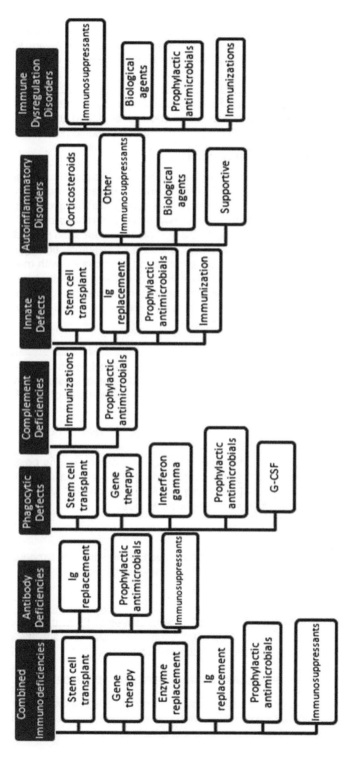

Fig. 3. Therapies for various types of primary immunodeficiencies. (*Data from* Refs. [16,17,19–26])

Autoinflammatory disorders can be treated depending on the etiopathogenesis. Corticosteroids can be used for some periodic fever syndromes. IL1 receptor antagonists such as anakinra can be used in inflammasome-associated periodic fevers. HSCT has been used for IL10 defects causing early-onset inflammatory bowel disease.

Symptomatic Treatment

Prompt recognition and treatment of infections and other complications is the key to keeping patients with PID healthy. Every effort should be made to obtain the microbiological diagnosis; however, institution of empiric therapy should not be delayed.

Prevention of Manifestations/Complications

Lifestyle changes to prevent infections and other complications can significantly improve morbidity of patients with PID. The importance of hand washing and overall hygiene cannot be overstated. Patients should be educated about avoiding sick contacts and unimmunized contacts. A discussion with the health care provider regarding immunization is important. Depending on the type of PID, patients can receive some or all of the routine immunizations; in particular, ensuring annual protection against influenza (ie, influenza vaccine) needs to be emphasized. Compliance with medications and office visits can play an important role in the care of these patients. A healthy lifestyle with nutritious diet and aerobic exercise is important to ensuring optimal quality of life. Along with the guidance on physical health, resources should be provided for maintaining mental and emotional well-being.

Follow-up/Monitoring

Regular follow-up with the primary care provider as well as the immunologist should be encouraged. Depending on the type of PID, interval laboratory evaluation and imaging should be used to monitor for the complications of the PID or its treatment.

PROGNOSIS

Discussions with the patient/family should include elaboration on the possible outcomes of the condition, including rare complications and complications of the treatment modalities. Although prognosis varies depending on the type of PID, the common factors affecting the overall prognosis include:

- Age at diagnosis
- Presence of infections
- Presence of noninfectious complications such as lung disease, lymphoproliferation, granulomatous disease, or autoimmune complications
- Age at the time of definitive treatment (eg, HSCT)
- Other comorbidities

With the advances in the discovery of genetic causes of PIDs, it is important to counsel families about the implications for future family planning and the patient's probability of passing on the defect to future generations.

FUTURE OF THE STUDY OF PRIMARY IMMUNODEFICIENCY DISORDERS

With rapidly improving genetic technology, the field of PIDs is expanding exponentially. As next-generation sequencing continues to reveal new defects, there is a growing need to improve the functional immunologic assays that uncover the underlying pathophysiology and molecular mechanisms.

Gene therapy, newer biologic agents, and possibly RNA interference therapies promise to dramatically improve outcomes for individuals with PIDs and their families.

REFERENCES

1. Ochs HD, Hitzig WH. History of primary immunodeficiency diseases. Curr Opin Allergy Clin Immunol 2012;12(6):577–87.
2. Al-Herz W, Bousfiha A, Casanova JL, et al. Primary immunodeficiency diseases: an update on the classification from the international union of immunological societies expert committee for primary immunodeficiency. Front Immunol 2014;5: 162.
3. Yel L. Selective IgA deficiency. J Clin Immunol 2010;30(1):10–6.
4. Kwan A, Abraham RS, Currier R, et al. Newborn screening for severe combined immunodeficiency in 11 screening programs in the United States. JAMA 2014; 312(7):729–38.
5. Routes J, Abinun M, Al-Herz W, et al. ICON: the early diagnosis of congenital immunodeficiencies. J Clin Immunol 2014;34(4):398–424.
6. Grumach AS, Kirschfink M. Are complement deficiencies really rare? Overview on prevalence, clinical importance and modern diagnostic approach. Mol Immunol 2014;61(2):110–7.
7. Picard C, Casanova JL, Puel A. Infectious diseases in patients with IRAK-4, MyD88, NEMO, or IkappaBalpha deficiency. Clin Microbiol Rev 2011;24(3):490–7.
8. Pannicke U, Baumann B, Fuchs S, et al. Deficiency of innate and acquired immunity caused by an IKBKB mutation. N Engl J Med 2013;369(26):2504–14.
9. Frazao JB, Errante PR, Condino-Neto A. Toll-like receptors' pathway disturbances are associated with increased susceptibility to infections in humans. Arch Immunol Ther Exp (Warsz) 2013;61(6):427–43.
10. Orange JS. Natural killer cell deficiency. J Allergy Clin Immunol 2013;132(3): 515–25 [quiz: 526].
11. Faitelson Y, Grunebaum E. Hemophagocytic lymphohistiocytosis and primary immune deficiency disorders. Clin Immunol 2014;155(1):118–25.
12. Charbonnier LM, Janssen E, Chou J, et al. Regulatory T-cell deficiency and immune dysregulation, polyendocrinopathy, enteropathy, X-linked-like disorder caused by loss-of-function mutations in LRBA. J Allergy Clin Immunol 2015; 135(1):217–27.
13. Verbsky JW, Chatila TA. Immune dysregulation, polyendocrinopathy, enteropathy, X-linked (IPEX) and IPEX-related disorders: an evolving web of heritable autoimmune diseases. Curr Opin Pediatr 2013;25(6):708–14.
14. Veillette A, Perez-Quintero LA, Latour S. X-linked lymphoproliferative syndromes and related autosomal recessive disorders. Curr Opin Allergy Clin Immunol 2013; 13(6):614–22.
15. Lohr NJ, Molleston JP, Strauss KA, et al. Human ITCH E3 ubiquitin ligase deficiency causes syndromic multisystem autoimmune disease. Am J Hum Genet 2010;86(3):447–53.
16. Oliveira JB, Bleesing JJ, Dianzani U, et al. Revised diagnostic criteria and classification for the autoimmune lymphoproliferative syndrome (ALPS): report from the 2009 NIH International Workshop. Blood 2010;116(14):e35–40.
17. Rigante D, Vitale A, Lucherini OM, et al. The hereditary autoinflammatory disorders uncovered. Autoimmun Rev 2014;13(9):892–900.
18. Locke BA, Dasu T, Verbsky JW. Laboratory diagnosis of primary immunodeficiencies. Clin Rev Allergy Immunol 2014;46(2):154–68.

19. Berger M. Choices in IgG replacement therapy for primary immune deficiency diseases: subcutaneous IgG vs. intravenous IgG and selecting an optimal dose. Curr Opin Allergy Clin Immunol 2011;11(6):532–8.

20. Verbsky JW, Routes JM. Sarcoidosis and common variable immunodeficiency: similarities and differences. Semin Respir Crit Care Med 2014;35(3):330–5.

21. Wehr C, Gennery AR, Lindemans C, et al. Multicenter experience in hematopoietic stem cell transplantation for serious complications of common variable immunodeficiency. J Allergy Clin Immunol 2015;135(4):988–97.e6.

22. Farinelli G, Capo V, Scaramuzza S, et al. Lentiviral vectors for the treatment of primary immunodeficiencies. J Inherit Metab Dis 2014;37(4):525–33.

23. Pai SY, Logan BR, Griffith LM, et al. Transplantation outcomes for severe combined immunodeficiency, 2000-2009. N Engl J Med 2014;371(5):434–46.

24. de la Morena MT, Nelson RP Jr. Recent advances in transplantation for primary immune deficiency diseases: a comprehensive review. Clin Rev Allergy Immunol 2014;46(2):131–44.

25. Jyonouchi S, McDonald-McGinn DM, Bale S, et al. CHARGE (coloboma, heart defect, atresia choanae, retarded growth and development, genital hypoplasia, ear anomalies/deafness) syndrome and chromosome 22q11.2 deletion syndrome: a comparison of immunologic and nonimmunologic phenotypic features. Pediatrics 2009;123(5):e871–7.

26. Gennery AR. Immunological aspects of 22q11.2 deletion syndrome. Cell Mol Life Sci 2012;69(1):17–27.

27. Stiehm RE, Ochs HD, Winkelstein JA. Immunodeficiency disorders: general considerations. 5th edition. Philadelphia (PA): Saunders; 2004.

28. Driessen G, van der Burg M. Educational paper: primary antibody deficiencies. Eur J Pediatr 2011;170(6):693–702.

29. Winkelstein JA, Marino MC, Lederman HM, et al. X-linked agammaglobulinemia: report on a United States registry of 201 patients. Medicine (Baltimore) 2006; 85(4):193–202.

30. Cunningham-Rundles C. The many faces of common variable immunodeficiency. Hematol Am Soc Hematol Educ Program 2012;2012:301–5.

31. Qamar N, Fuleihan RL. The hyper IgM syndromes. Clin Rev Allergy Immunol 2014;46(2):120–30.

32. Winkelstein JA, Marino MC, Ochs H, et al. The X-linked hyper-IgM syndrome: clinical and immunologic features of 79 patients. Medicine (Baltimore) 2003;82(6): 373–84.

33. Crank MC, Grossman JK, Moir S, et al. Mutations in PIK3CD can cause hyper IgM syndrome (HIGM) associated with increased cancer susceptibility. J Clin Immunol 2014;34(3):272–6.

34. Picard C, Dogniaux S, Chemin K, et al. Hypomorphic mutation of ZAP70 in human results in a late onset immunodeficiency and no autoimmunity. Eur J Immunol 2009;39(7):1966–76.

35. de la Calle-Martin O, Hernandez M, Ordi J, et al. Familial CD8 deficiency due to a mutation in the CD8 alpha gene. J Clin Invest 2001;108(1):117–23.

36. Zimmer J, Andres E, Donato L, et al. Clinical and immunological aspects of HLA class I deficiency. QJM 2005;98(10):719–27.

37. Reith W, Mach B. The bare lymphocyte syndrome and the regulation of MHC expression. Annu Rev Immunol 2001;19:331–73.

38. Li FY, Lenardo MJ, Chaigne-Delalande B. Loss of MAGT1 abrogates the Mg2+ flux required for T cell signaling and leads to a novel human primary immunodeficiency. Magnesium Res 2011;24(3):S109–14.

39. Hauck F, Randriamampita C, Martin E, et al. Primary T-cell immunodeficiency with immunodysregulation caused by autosomal recessive LCK deficiency. J Allergy Clin Immunol 2012;130(5):1144–52.e11.
40. Lopez-Herrera G, Tampella G, Pan-Hammarstrom Q, et al. Deleterious mutations in LRBA are associated with a syndrome of immune deficiency and autoimmunity. Am J Hum Genet 2012;90(6):986–1001.
41. Gorska MM, Alam R. A mutation in the human Uncoordinated 119 gene impairs TCR signaling and is associated with CD4 lymphopenia. Blood 2012;119(6): 1399–406.
42. van Montfrans JM, Hoepelman AI, Otto S, et al. CD27 deficiency is associated with combined immunodeficiency and persistent symptomatic EBV viremia. J Allergy Clin Immunol 2012;129(3):787–93.e6.
43. Ghosh S, Bienemann K, Boztug K, et al. Interleukin-2-inducible T-cell kinase (ITK) deficiency - clinical and molecular aspects. J Clin Immunol 2014;34(8):892–9.
44. Buchbinder D, Nugent DJ, Fillipovich AH. Wiskott-Aldrich syndrome: diagnosis, current management, and emerging treatments. Appl Clin Genet 2014;7:55–66.
45. Lanzi G, Moratto D, Vairo D, et al. A novel primary human immunodeficiency due to deficiency in the WASP-interacting protein WIP. J Exp Med 2012;209(1):29–34.
46. O'Driscoll M. Diseases associated with defective responses to DNA damage. Cold Spring Harb Perspect Biol 2012;4(12) [pii:a012773].
47. Baradaran-Heravi A, Thiel C, Rauch A, et al. Clinical and genetic distinction of Schimke immuno-osseous dysplasia and cartilage-hair hypoplasia. Am J Med Genet A 2008;146A(15):2013–7.
48. Farmand S, Sundin M. Hyper-IgE syndromes: recent advances in pathogenesis, diagnostics and clinical care. Curr Opin Hematol 2015;22(1):12–22.
49. Etzioni A. Genetic etiologies of leukocyte adhesion defects. Curr Opin Immunol 2009;21(5):481–6.
50. Hsu AP, McReynolds LJ, Holland SM. GATA2 deficiency. Curr Opin Allergy Clin Immunol 2015;15(1):104–9.

Approach to Children with Recurrent Infections

Vivian P. Hernandez-Trujillo, MD[a,b,*]

KEYWORDS

- Recurrent infections • Children • Immunodeficiency • Pediatric • Recurrent fever

KEY POINTS

- Frequent infections are common in young children, especially on first exposure to the day care or school setting.
- Severe infections that do not respond to traditional treatment can indicate a more serious underlying disorder of the immune system.
- Infections that are severe, persistent, unusual, or recurrent should be red flags to alert clinicians about patients who should have an immune work-up.
- Screening immune laboratory tests may be done initially, followed by a work-up guided by the type of infections, along with microorganism susceptibility.
- Prompt diagnosis and treatment are essential in minimizing the long-term effects from recurrent infections.

INTRODUCTION

Young children often present with a history of recurrent infections, especially once they are introduced to the day care or school setting. Children who present with recurrent infections before this introduction are even more concerning, particularly in children with failure to thrive or recurrent diarrhea. The childhood presentation of primary immunodeficiency diseases is common, although often misdiagnosed. Clinicians need to keep primary immunodeficiency in the differential diagnosis when caring for children who present with recurrent infections, particularly sinopulmonary infections. Campaigns have been created by the Immune Deficiency Foundation (IDF) and the

Disclosure: Advisory Board for Baxter Pharmaceuticals, CSL Behring, and Merck/Bayer; speakers bureau for Baxter Pharmaceuticals, CSL Behring; attendee at International Immune Globulin Conference, CSL Behring; research grant recipient, CSL Behring.

[a] Division of Allergy and Immunology, Department of Pediatrics, Nicklaus Children's Hospital, 3100 Southwest 62 Avenue, Miami, FL 33155, USA; [b] Herbert Wertheim School of Medicine, Florida International University, Miami, FL 33199, USA
* Division of Allergy and Immunology, Nicklaus Children's Hospital, 3100 Southwest 62 Avenue, Miami, FL 33155.
E-mail address: Vivian.Hernandez-Trujillo@mch.com

Immunol Allergy Clin N Am 35 (2015) 625–636
http://dx.doi.org/10.1016/j.iac.2015.07.005   immunology.theclinics.com

Jeffrey Modell Foundation (JMF) to increase awareness regarding the diagnosis of primary immunodeficiency diseases.[1,2]

SYMPTOMS/SIGNS

Patients with recurrent episodes of febrile illness may initially present with infections in any organ system.[3] Most commonly, viral infections cause recurrent fever in young children.[3] Although the most common presentation includes the sinopulmonary tract, infections can occur in any other organ system, commonly the gastrointestinal or mucocutaneous systems.[4] If febrile episodes occur within specific time periods (ie, every week to 3 weeks), other diagnoses, such as periodic fever syndromes or cyclic neutropenia, should be considered.[3]

Recurrent sinopulmonary infections are a common hallmark in patients with recurrent infections. Recent studies show the role of CD4+ T-helper lymphocytes in protection against common organisms, such as *Streptococcus pneumoniae* and *Haemophilus influenzae*.[5] Pediatric patients with frequent otitis media (OM) infections were more likely to have lower levels of pneumococcal-specific immunoglobulin (Ig) G, as well as lower *S pneumoniae*–specific memory B cells, compared with children not prone to OM. Importantly, these patients also had lower levels of major histocompatibility complex II molecules on the surface of dendritic cells, which are potent antigen-presenting cells.[5] These children, prone to OM, had poor responses to more than half the vaccine antigens studied. Children with frequent OM also had lower increases in antibodies between the ages of 6 and 24 months to *S pneumoniae* compared with children not prone to OM. [5]

Patients with recurrent infections may have other related disease, either gastrointestinal or respiratory. In some patients with recurrent OM, gastroesophageal reflux (GERD) is likely to play a role.[6] Pepsin/pepsinogen was found in the middle ear of these patients, which may be related to GERD. The investigators found that GERD prevalence may be higher in patients with recurrent OM or chronic OM with effusion. In another study, structural airway abnormalities may have contributed to recurrent lower respiratory tract infections.[7] In that study, 50% of children with lower respiratory tract infections also had tracheomalacia and/or bronchomalacia. Patients more often had positive bronchoalveolar lavage cultures to nontypable *H influenzae* or *S pneumoniae*.[7]

In children, urinary tract infections are the second most common bacterial infection.[8] Urothelium expresses toll-like receptors that, when engaged, can result in inflammation, potentially leading to damage of the kidneys.[8] A recent study in patients with vesicoureteral reflux showed that antimicrobial prophylaxis decreased the risk of recurrence of urinary tract infections.[9] Patients with bladder and bowel dysfunction with index febrile infection benefited from antibiotic prophylaxis.[10] Patients with recurrent infections of a particular location in the body (eg, urinary tract infections) may have deficiency of the innate or complement system (**Fig. 1**). Toll-like receptor 4 (TLR4) is essential in a patient's susceptibility to urinary tract infections.[10] Patients with asymptomatic bacteriuria differed from those prone to recurrent acute pyelonephritis in that they had lower TLR4 expression in response to infection, suggesting that this attenuates the innate response at the mucosal level.[10]

Pediatric patients often present with group A streptococcus pharyngitis infections, and clinicians should consider whether the patient may be a carrier when the infections are recurrent. Treatment of carrier state may be helpful, whereas other patients may require tonsillectomy. One study compared children with recurrent community-acquired pneumonia that affected different lung areas with children who never had

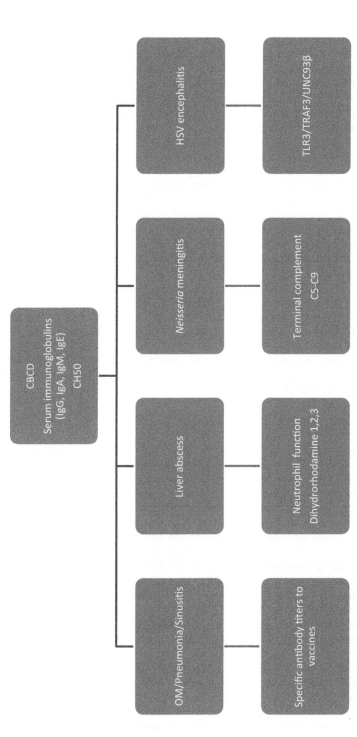

Fig. 1. Some primary immunodeficiencies can be diagnosed via a laboratory workup based on the site of infection. CH50, total complement hemolytic activity; HSV, herpes simplex virus; TLR3, toll-like receptor 3; TRAF3, tumor necrosis factor receptor–associated factor 3.

pneumonia.[11] The patients with recurrent community-acquired pneumonia were more likely to be premature, to have lower birth weight, to have a history of respiratory distress at birth, and to have started day care at an earlier age than control patients.[11] The investigators also described risk factors that are associated with community-acquired pneumonia recurrences, which include asthma, recurrent upper respiratory infections, atopy, chronic rhinosinusitis with postnasal drip, and wheezing.[11]

Depending on the types of infections, presenting signs and symptoms may vary. Patients with recurrent fungal or viral infections may present with failure to thrive or chronic diarrhea.[12] Other patients may present with lymphadenitis or abscesses, which may be recurrent and severe. Still other patients may have difficulty with neisseria meningitis or recurrent infections caused by encapsulated organisms. Each of these presentations leads to a different diagnostic work-up.[12]

A campaign regarding the types of infections that should be red flags for patients with recurrent infections exists through the IDF.[1] Children with recurrent infections that are severe, persistent, unusual, recurrent, or that run in the family should be considered for a work-up for primary immunodeficiency. When an infection is severe, does not respond to traditional antibiotic or antifungal treatment, is unusual or recurrent, or is present in family members, laboratory tests should be ordered to investigate the immune system.

Criteria have also been developed by the JMF for warning signs that the immune system may be faulty (**Box 1**).[2] The criteria are important reminders of signs that may indicate defects in the patient's immune system. The number of ear or sinus infections within a year and the number of deep infections, such as abscesses or sepsis, are some of the warning signs. The need for intravenous antibiotics to clear infections is another criterion. Failure of children to gain weight and weight loss in adults are also important signs of possible immunodeficiency. A family history of primary immunodeficiency (PI) is also one of the criteria.

DIAGNOSTIC TEST/IMAGING STUDY

A basic immune screening includes a complete blood count with differential (CBCD) (**Box 2**). More extensive studies depend on the types of infections the child has had. In patients with recurrent bacterial infections, such as sinopulmonary infections like OM, sinusitis, or pneumonia, serum immunoglobulin levels (IgG, IgA, IgM, IgE) are an important screening tool.[12] In young children who have not received vaccines, isohemagglutinins may provide information regarding antibody function. More extensive studies to investigate antibody function are specific antibody levels to vaccines, such as diphtheria, tetanus, H influenzae type B, or S pneumoniae titers.[12,13]

Administration of vaccines is a way to assess the patients' ability to produce antibodies.[13] For assessment of protein antibody production, levels of antibodies to diphtheria and tetanus can be measured. For assessment of polysaccharide antibody production, levels of antibodies to H influenzae type B and S pneumoniae can be measured postvaccine, 4 weeks after the vaccine administration. In general, a 2-fold response compared with prevaccination titers is considered an adequate response to vaccination. If the titers are protective before vaccination, significant increases are less likely.[13] Sometimes patients have an adequate antibody response with decreased clinical infections, but patients may develop recurrent infections after some time has passed from the vaccine administration.[13] Because antibody levels decrease over time in healthy individuals, administration of a vaccine and assessment of the antibody response can help distinguish patients with immune defects from those with normal waning titers.

Box 1
JMF: 10 warning signs of primary immunodeficiency (PI)

Pediatrics

1. Four or more new ear infections within 1 year

2. Two or more serious sinus infections within 1 year

3. Two or more months on antibiotics with little effect

4. Two or more pneumonias within 1 year

5. Failure of an infant to gain weight or grow normally

6. Recurrent deep skin or organ abscesses

7. Persistent thrush in mouth or fungal infection on skin

8. Need for intravenous antibiotics to clear infections

9. Two or more deep-seated infections including septicemia

10. A family history of PI

Adults

1. Two or more new ear infections within 1 year

2. Two or more new sinus infections within 1 year, in the absence of allergy

3. One pneumonia per year for more than 1 year

4. Chronic diarrhea with weight loss

5. Recurrent viral infections (colds, herpes, warts, condyloma)

6. Recurrent need for intravenous antibiotics to clear infections

7. Recurrent, deep abscesses of the skin or internal organs

8. Persistent thrush or fungal infection on skin or elsewhere

9. Infection with normally harmless tuberculosis-like bacteria

10. A family history of PI

These warning signs were developed by the Jeffrey Modell Foundation Medical Advisory Board. Consultation with primary immunodeficiency experts is strongly suggested. ©2009 Jeffrey Modell Foundation.

In patients with recurrent viral or fungal infections, the cellular immune system should be studied, including CBCD with special focus on absolute lymphocyte numbers, as well as lymphocyte enumeration (T, B, natural killer lymphocytes).[12] If these numbers are decreased, further laboratory investigation that assesses lymphocyte function, including proliferation to mitogens, should be ordered. In patients with recurrent lymphadenitis or abscess formation, neutrophil function should be evaluated with dihydrorhodamine 1,2,3 or oxidative burst. Patients with neisseria meningitis should be evaluated for complement deficiency with total complement hemolytic activity level (CH50).[12]

Box 2
General immune screening tests for recurrent infections

Complete blood count with differential

Serum immunoglobulins (IgG, IgA, IgM, IgE)

Total complement hemolytic activity

In some patients, the site of the infection or the microorganism responsible for the infections aids the clinician in deciding which part of the immune system should be studied further[14] (see **Fig. 1**; **Fig. 2**, **Table 1**). In patients with recurrent meningococcal infections, terminal complement levels (C5–C9) are helpful. Patients with recurrent salmonella or atypical mycobacterial infection may have deficiency of interleukin (IL) 12β receptor or interferon gamma receptor,[15] whereas those with recurrent pneumococcal infections may have deficiency of IL1 receptor–associated kinase 4 (IRAK4) or mutations in toll-like receptor 3 (TLR3), TRAF3 (tumor necrosis factor receptor–associated factor 3), and UNC93β (UNC-93 homolog B1 [C elegans]) genes.[14,16] Recurrent candida infections may be a clue that there is a susceptibility caused by a PI, with many possible defects responsible for the susceptibility (including STAT1, STAT3, IL17RA, IL17F, CARD9 [caspase recruitment domain member 9], dectin 1, IL22, IL12Rβ).[17,18] Chronic mucocutaneous candidiasis has presentations that vary from being alone to presenting as part of a syndrome, such as autoimmune polyendocrinopathy candidiasis ectodermal dystrophy or hyper-IgE syndrome (HIES).[17,19] In contrast, patients with persistent and symptomatic Epstein-Barr virus viremia may have CD27 deficiency.[20] Patients with problems caused by recurrent warts and hypogammaglobulinemia may have WHIM (warts, hypogammaglobulinemia, infections, and myelokathexis) syndrome,[21] whereas those with monocytopenia and *Mycobacterium avium* complex may have MonoMac syndrome, and thus deficiency of Gata binding protein 2 (GATA-2) should be considered.[22]

DIFFERENTIAL DIAGNOSIS

Some patients with recurrent OM have specific congenital disorders that are associated with recurrent OM.[23] These primary immunodeficiencies encompass different parts of the immune system, including diseases that affect antibody production, cellular disorders, and phagocytic disorders. Examples include X-linked agammaglobulinemia (XLA), common variable immunodeficiency (CVID), hyper-IgM syndrome, DiGeorge syndrome, ataxia telangiectasia, Wiskott-Aldrich syndrome, HIES, and chronic granulomatous disease (CGD).[23] These diseases should be kept in mind when assessing patients with recurrent OM.

Children may present with recurrent infections caused by other systemic diseases (**Box 3**). Gastroesophageal reflux that is severe can also lead to recurrent infections, both upper respiratory and OM.[6] In children with a history of failure to thrive, poor weight gain, respiratory infections, and diarrhea, cystic fibrosis (CF) should be considered. Recurrent lung infections, particularly from *Pseudomonas aeruginosa* and *Staphylococcus aureus*, lead to loss in pulmonary function, and thus damage to the lungs.[24] Early diagnosis in the first 5 years of life, especially before the patients become symptomatic, is essential in preventing progressive lung disease. Screening tests, such as a sweat test or genetic testing, are available to screen for and diagnose CF. Other diseases to consider include ciliary dyskinesia, which can lead to recurrent sinopulmonary infections.[25] These patients present with recurrent OM or sinusitis that does not improve despite antibiotic treatment. Patients develop bronchiectasis. Some patients with ciliary dyskinesia have humoral immunodeficiency, and many have difficulties with *P aeruginosa* infections.[25] Ciliary biopsy can be done to aid in the diagnosis of this disease. Other patients, with diseases like alpha1-antitrypsin deficiency, present with recurrent respiratory infections like pneumonia, bleeding disorders, and liver disease.[26] The initial presentation may include respiratory symptoms, such as cough and shortness of breath. Later, the patients frequently develop emphysema and liver failure. Levels of alpha1-antitrypsin can be measured, followed by phenotype and genotype screening.[26,27]

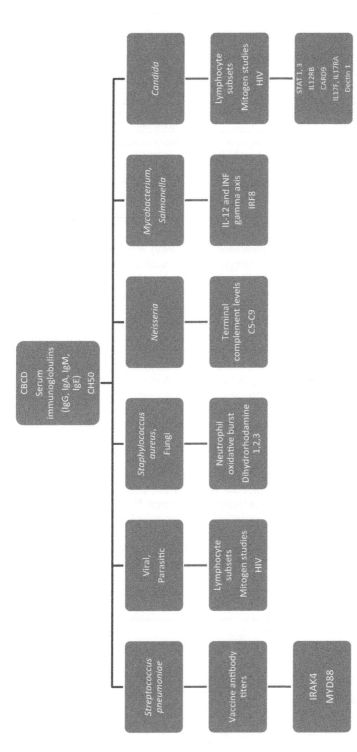

Fig. 2. Primary immunodeficiencies may present because of infections caused by specific microorganisms. In these patients, screening laboratory tests can be done, followed by work-up based on the organism and, in some cases, the genetic mutation leading to the infection. CARD9, caspase recruitment domain member 9; HIV, human immunodeficiency virus; IL, interleukin; INF, interferon; IRAK4, IL1 receptor–associated kinase 1; IRF8, interferon regulatory factor 8; MYD88, myeloid differentiation primary response gene 88; STAT, signal transducer and activation of transcription.

Table 1
Laboratory work-up based on location/type of infection and microorganism susceptibility

CBCD, serum immunoglobulins Specific antibody to vaccines	Sinopulmonary	S pneumoniae, Haemophilus influenzae type B, Enterovirus
CBCD, lymphocyte subsets	Varies	Viruses, fungi, Candida, Atypical mycobacterium, Pneumocystis jiroveci
CBCD, serum immunoglobulins Lymphocyte subsets	Sinopulmonary	Bacteria, viruses, fungi, P jiroveci, parasites
CBCD, oxidative burst	Abscesses, lymphadenitis	Staphylococcus aureus, Salmonella, Nocardia, atypical mycobacteria Fungi: Aspergillus
Total complement	Meningitis	Streptococcus, H influenza type B, Neisseria

Patients with human immunodeficiency virus (HIV) also frequently present with recurrent infections, often viral or fungal. Children with congenital HIV may present with opportunistic infections.[28] Mothers infected with HIV have lower transplacental antibody transfer than mothers without HIV. In children without known HIV diagnosis, opportunistic infections are often the presenting symptom. In these children, maternally transferred antibodies can complicate the diagnosis of some infections.[28] Antiretroviral therapy helps within the first few months of treatment, and is important in improving CD4 counts and immune function. Patients who responded to highly active antiretroviral therapy (HAART) were more likely to have opportunistic infections and herpes zoster, Cytomegalovirus, and herpes simplex before HAART.[29] This finding is another reminder of the importance of proper diagnosis, as early as possible to ensure proper treatment.

TREATMENT

When patients have defects in antibody production, such as in XLA, CVID, hyper-IgM syndrome, and others, immune globulin replacement, available via intravenous and subcutaneous administration, is the treatment of choice.[30] Some patients also benefit from prophylactic antibiotics.[12] Patients with cellular defects may benefit from aggressive antibiotic treatment of infections or prophylaxis with antibiotics.[12] In contrast, some patients with complete DiGeorge syndrome/22q11 deletion benefit from thymic transplant.[31] Patients with defective combined antibody and cellular defects, such as severe combined immunodeficiency, need more aggressive treatment, including immune globulin replacement, leading to stem cell transplant. Proper nutrition,

Box 3
Differential diagnosis in children with recurrent infections

Cystic fibrosis

Ciliary dyskinesia

Alpha1-antitrypsin deficiency

Gastroesophageal reflux

Human immunodeficiency virus (HIV1, HIV2)

aggressive treatment of infections, and prophylactic antibiotics are important in protecting the patients until they are able to receive their transplants.[32]

Some patients with neutrophil disorders, like CGD, benefit from stem cell transplant, whereas others benefit from treatment with prophylaxis with itraconazole and trimethoprim/sulfamethoxazole.[33,34] The use of gamma interferon to improve oxidative burst in these patients is also of benefit. Some newer studies are investigating gene therapy for these patients.[35,36] Patients with terminal complement deficiency also benefit from prophylaxis with penicillin.[12]

For patients with CF, inhaled nebulized hypertonic saline, used to increase mucociliary clearance, along with antibiotic therapy, such as macrolide antibiotics, are important for the treatment of infections that can damage the lung, as well as for breaking up mucus.[24] Patients also benefit from chest physical therapy. Patients with ciliary dyskinesia should be treated aggressively with antibiotics, chest physical therapy and bronchodilators, and antiinflammatory medications.[25] Patients with alpha1-antitrypsin may require organ transplant for progressive lung or liver disease.[26] Some patients with Pi ZZ phenotype and forced expiratory volume in 1 second less than 65% benefit from intravenous alpha1-antitrypsin. Long-acting bronchodilators and inhaled corticosteroids are important in the treatment of the lung disease.[26] Influenza vaccinations yearly and pneumococcal vaccines every 5 years are also recommended. Patients with HIV can benefit from early combination retroviral therapy or HAART.[28,29] Patients treated with HAART had few opportunistic infections.[29]

MANAGEMENT

Long-term management should include careful monitoring by the primary care physician, along with the specialist, whether immunologist, pulmonologist, or gastroenterologist, depending on the disease responsible for the recurrent infections. The management is necessary in order to assess whether any change has occurred that may necessitate treatment, and to ensure that the patients are responding to therapy appropriately, if they are on a treatment plan.

Good nutrition, sleep, and exercise are also recommendations that are likely to benefit most patients with recurrent infections. Recommendations for overall maintenance of health may be useful, including regular use of hand washing, barrier techniques, and exercise. Use of hygiene measures has been shown to help prevent the spread of infections, both respiratory and gastrointestinal.[36–40] Prevention of the spread of influenza has been seen with the use of face masks with hand hygiene in both home and community settings.[36,37] Alcohol-based rub, foam, and wipes helped reduce the amount of virus from hands.[38] Moderate exercise has been shown to improve immune response to viral respiratory tract infections.[41] The study also showed decreased inflammation from moderate exercise. Exercise also improves the immune response of the innate system.[42] These recommendations are important for the overall health of the patients.

Interest in the use of probiotics in patients with recurrent infections has also grown. A recent meta-analysis found that probiotics were beneficial, compared with placebo, for prevention of recurrent infections.[43] The patients treated with probiotics had less antibiotic use and fewer episodes of acute upper respiratory tract infection. However, in some populations, the risk of sepsis exists if patients take probiotics, in particular in immunocompromised patients or premature infants.[43] Studies are needed regarding the use of probiotics in the treatment of upper respiratory tract infections.

Depending on the underlying disease that leads to recurrent infections, comanagement by the primary care physician and a specialist, either immunology for PI or pulmonology and gastroenterology for CF or alpha1-antitrypsin deficiency, may be most helpful in attaining the best outcomes for the patients. Genetic counseling for patients who have a congenital or hereditary disease is also recommended.

SUMMARY

The approach to patients with recurrent infections should begin with a thorough history and physician examination, followed by screening laboratory tests. The types of infections, sites of infection, and microorganisms leading to infection are also helpful in guiding clinicians as to which parts of the immune system should be further studied. Immunology knowledge continues to expand, as new genetic diagnoses are added to the list of primary immunodeficiencies.[44,45] The differential also includes common diseases that should be considered in patients with recurrent infections. Treatment should be targeted toward the particular disease that is causing the recurrent infections. Long-term management is essential in ensuring the health of any patient with chronic disease, in particular PI.

REFERENCES

1. Marshall GS. Prolonged and recurrent fevers in children. J Infect 2014;68:583–93.
2. Lehman H, Hernandez-Trujillo V, Ballow M. Diagnosing primary immunodeficiency: a practical approach for the non-immunologist. Curr Med Res Opin 2015;31:1–10.
3. Immune Deficiency Foundation. Available at: http://primaryimmune.org/wp-content/uploads/2014/09/InfoCard.pdf. Accessed March 11, 2015.
4. Jeffrey Modell Foundation. Available at: http://www.info4pi.org/library/educational-materials. Accessed March 11, 2015.
5. Sharma SK, Pichichero ME. Cellular immune responses in young children accounts for recurrent acute otitis media. Curr Allergy Asthma Rep 2013;13:495–500.
6. Miura MS, Mascaro M, Rosenfeld RM. Association between otitis media and gastroesophageal reflux: a systematic review. Otolaryngol Head Neck Surg 2012;146:345–52.
7. Santiago-Burruchaga M, Zalacain-Jorge R, Vazquez-Cordero C. Are airways structural abnormalities more frequent in children with recurrent lower respiratory tract infections? Respir Med 2014;108:800–5.
8. Mak RH, Kuo HJ. Pathogenesis of urinary tract infection: an update. Curr Opin Pediatr 2006;18:148–52.
9. RIVUR Trial Investigators. Antimicrobial prophylaxis for children with vesicoureteral reflux. N Engl J Med 2014;370:2367–76.
10. Ragnarsdottir B, Jonsson K, Urbano A, et al. Toll-like receptor 4 promoter polymorphisms: common TLR4 variants may protect against severe urinary tract infection. PLoS One 2010;5:e10734.
11. Patria F, Longhi B, Tagliabue C, et al. Clinical profile of recurrent community-acquired pneumonia in children. BMC Pulm Med 2013;13:60–8.
12. Bonilla FA, Bernstein IL, Khan DA, et al. Practice parameter for the diagnosis and management of primary immunodeficiency. Ann Allergy Asthma Immunol 2005;94:S1–63.
13. Ballow M. Use of vaccines in the evaluation of presumed immunodeficiency. Ann Allergy Asthma Immunol 2013;111:163–6.
14. Notarangelo LD. Primary immunodeficiencies. J Allergy Clin Immunol 2010;125(2 Suppl 2):S182–94.

15. Hambleton S, Salem S, Bustamante J, et al. Mutations in IRF8 and human dendritic cell immunodeficiency. N Engl J Med 2011;365:127–38.

16. Picard C, Casanova JL, Puel A. Infectious diseases in patients with IRAK-4, MyD88, NEMO or Iκβα deficiency. Clin Microbiol Rev 2011;24:490–7.

17. Kisand K, Peterson P. Autoimmune polyendocrinopathy candidiasis ectodermal dystrophy and other primary immunodeficiency diseases help to resolve the nature of protective immunity against chronic mucocutaneous candidiasis. Curr Opin Pediatr 2013;25(6):715–21.

18. Puel A, Cypowyj S, Buatamante J, et al. Chronic mucocutaneous candidiasis in humans with inborn errors of interleukin-17 immunity. Science 2011;332:65–8.

19. Zhang Q, Su HC. Hyperimmunoglobulin E syndromes in pediatrics. Curr Opin Pediatr 2011;23:653–8.

20. Van Montfrans JM, Hoepelman AI, Otto S, et al. CD27 deficiency is associated with combined immunodeficiency and persistent symptomatic EBV viremia. J Allergy Clin Immunol 2012;129:787–93.

21. Tassone L, Notorangelo LD, Bonomi V, et al. Clinical and genetic diagnosis of warts, hypogammaglobulinemia, infections and myelokathexis syndrome in 10 patients. J Allergy Clin Immunol 2009;123:1170–3.

22. Bigley V, Collin M. Dendritic cell, monocyte, B and NK lymphoid deficiency defines the lost lineages of a new GATA-2 dependent myelodysplastic syndrome. Haematologica 2011;96:1081–3.

23. Urschel S. Otitis media children with congenital immunodeficiencies. Curr Allergy Asthma Rep 2010;10:425–33.

24. Grasemann H, Ratjen F. Early lung disease in cystic fibrosis. Lancet Respir Med 2013;1:148–57.

25. Boon M, De Boeck K, Jorissen M, et al. Primary ciliary dyskinesia and humoral immunodeficiency–Is there a missing link? Respir Med 2014;108:931–4.

26. Fregonese L, Stolk J. Hereditary alpha-1-antitrypsin deficiency and its clinical consequences. Orphanet J Rare Dis 2008;3:16–25.

27. Aboussouan LS, Stoller JK. Detection of alpha-1-antitrypsin deficiency: a review. Respir Med 2009;103:335–41.

28. Siberry GK, Abzug MJ, Nachman S, et al. Guidelines for the prevention and treatment of opportunistic infections in HIV-exposed and HIV-infected children. Pediatr Infect Dis J 2013;32:1–10.

29. Nesheim SR, Hardnett F, Wheeling JT, et al. Incidence of opportunistic illness before and after initiation of highly active antiretroviral therapy in children in LEGACY. Pediatr Infect Dis J 2013;32:1089–95.

30. Orange JS, Hossny EM, Weiler CR, et al. Use of intravenous immunoglobulin in human disease: a review of evidence by members of the Primary Immunodeficiency Committee of the Academy of Allergy, Asthma and Immunology. J Allergy Clin Immunol 2006;117:S525–53.

31. Markert ML, Devlin BH, McCarthy EA. Thymus transplantation. Clin Immunol 2010;135(2):236–46.

32. Cossu F. Genetics of SCID. Ital J Pediatr 2010;36:76–93.

33. Freeman AF, Holland SM. Antimicrobial prophylaxis for primary immunodeficiencies. Curr Opin Allergy Clin Immunol 2009;9(6):525–30.

34. Kaufmann KB, Chiriaco M, Siler U, et al. Gene therapy for chronic granulomatous disease: current status and future perspectives. Curr Gene Ther 2014;14(6):447–60.

35. Griffith LM, Cowan MJ, Notarangelo LD, et al, workshop participants. Primary Immune Deficiency Treatment Consortium (PIDTC) report. J Allergy Clin Immunol 2014;133(2):335–47.

36. Cowling BJ, Chan KH, Fang VJ, et al. Facemasks and hand hygiene to prevent influenza transmission in households: a cluster randomized trial. Ann Intern Med 2009;151:437–46.
37. Wong VW, Cowling BJ, Aiello AE. Hand hygiene and risk of influenza virus infections in the community: a systematic review and meta-analysis. Epidemiol Infect 2014;142(5):922–32.
38. Larson EL, Cohen B, Baxter KA. Analysis of alcohol-based hand sanitizer delivery systems: efficacy of foam, gel, and wipes against influenza A (H1N1) virus on hands. Am J Infect Control 2012;40(9):806–9.
39. Jefferson T, Del Mar C, Dooley L, et al. Physical interventions to interrupt or reduce the spread of respiratory viruses. Cochrane Database Syst Rev 2010;(7):CD006207.
40. Sandora TJ, Shih MC, Goldmann DA. Reducing absenteeism from gastrointestinal and respiratory illness in elementary school students: a randomized, controlled trial of an infection-control intervention. Pediatrics 2008;121:e1555–62.
41. Martin SA, Pence BD, Woods JA. Exercise and respiratory tract viral infections. Exerc Sport Sci Rev 2009;37(4):157–64.
42. Woods JA, Vieira VJ, Keylock KT. Exercise, inflammation, and innate immunity. Immunol Allergy Clin North Am 2009;29:381–93.
43. Esposito S, Rigante D, Principi N. Do children's upper respiratory tract infections benefit from probiotics? BMC Infect Dis 2014;14:194–201.
44. Al-Herz W, Bousfiha A, Casanova JL, et al. Primary immunodeficiency diseases: an update on the classification from the International Union of Immunological Societies Expert Committee for Primary Immunodeficiency. Front Immunol 2014;5:1–33.
45. Hernandez-Trujillo V. New genetic discoveries and primary immune deficiencies. Clin Rev Allergy Immunol 2014;46(2):145–53.

Common Variable Immunodeficiency

Diagnosis, Management, and Treatment

Jordan K. Abbott, MA, MD*, Erwin W. Gelfand, MD

KEYWORDS

- Common variable immunodeficiency • CVID • Antibody deficiency
- Primary immune deficiency • Immune activation • Autoimmunity
- Lymphoproliferation

KEY POINTS

- Common variable immunodeficiency (CVID) is a grouping of heterogeneous diseases with the common finding of impaired antibody production.
- Morbidity is not limited to infection; in fact, noninfectious complications can be the most threatening and difficult to treat.
- Proper care of patients with CVID includes both replacement of immunoglobulin G and monitoring for CVID-associated disease on a regular basis.

INTRODUCTION

Common variable immunodeficiency (CVID) refers to a grouping of antibody deficiencies that lack a more specific genetic or phenotypic classification. It is the immunodeficiency classification with the greatest number of constituents, likely because of the numerous ways in which antibody production can be impaired and the frequency in which antibody production becomes impaired in human beings. CVID comprises a heterogeneous group of rare diseases. Consequently, CVID presents a significant challenge for researchers and clinicians. Despite these difficulties, both our understanding of and ability to manage this grouping of complex immune diseases has advanced significantly over the past 60 years.

Disclaimers: none.
Division of Allergy and Immunology, Department of Pediatrics, National Jewish Health, 1400 Jackson Street, Denver, CO 80206, USA
* Corresponding author.
E-mail address: abbottj@njhealth.org

Immunol Allergy Clin N Am 35 (2015) 637–658
http://dx.doi.org/10.1016/j.iac.2015.07.009
0889-8561/15/$ – see front matter © 2015 Elsevier Inc. All rights reserved.

DIAGNOSIS
Initial Evaluation

Historically, the definition of common variable immunodeficiency (CVID) focused on the predominant finding of antibody deficiency, but more recent definitions have focused on the associated clinical features frequently seen. The most cited definition of CVID was presented by the European Society for Immunodeficiency (ESID) and the Pan American Group for Immunodeficiency in 1999, and the following criteria for probable CVID were proposed: greater than 2 years of age, immunoglobulin G (IgG) and immunoglobulin A (IgA) less than 2 standard deviations from the mean for age, either absent isohemagglutinin or absent vaccine responses, and no other defined causes of hypogammaglobulinemia.[1] Recently, there has been a growing concern that the application of these criteria to the clinical setting has resulted in the inappropriate administration of immunoglobulin replacement in a substantial number of patients that were unlikely to benefit from this therapy but still met the CVID criteria.[2] As a result, alternative diagnostic criteria have been proposed to include the following additional features: symptoms directly attributable to failure of antibody production, additional supportive laboratory findings, and pathologic confirmation of diseases frequently seen in CVID.[3] The latest combined ESID working criteria for classification of primary immune deficiency incorporated these concerns and also made efforts to remove diseases in which hypogammaglobulinemia likely results from a profound deficiency of T cells (**Table 1**).[1,4]

Differential Diagnosis

Secondary causes of decreased serum immunoglobulin levels must be ruled out in any patient that meets the diagnostic criteria for CVID because these causes can have dramatically different treatment implications. Infection, protein losing enteropathy, renal protein loss, genetic syndromes, immunosuppressive medications, other medications, and malignancy can all induce hypogammaglobulinemia.[2,5] Malignancy in particular can present with profound immune system derangement, and some advocate that all initial CVID diagnoses should remain provisional for a brief period of time to allow for emergence of malignancy.[3,6] Secondary causes of hypogammaglobulinemia are numerous, and the process of exclusion is often tedious; however, diligent consideration of these processes is essential to achieve an accurate diagnosis.

Pitfalls

The antibody response to polysaccharide pneumococcus vaccine, PNEUMOVAX23, is frequently measured to fulfill the antibody response criterion of the CVID diagnostic criteria; however, the validity of this type of testing is uncertain. In the United States, response to pneumococcal vaccination is assessed with laboratory-developed tests that demonstrate significant variability when the same sera are evaluated in different laboratories.[7] Additionally, what constitutes a normal response to vaccination lacks consensus; the chosen thresholds for measuring responsiveness dramatically influence the outcome.[8] Functional assays that measure opsonophagocytosis or antibody affinity promise to more accurately assess whether a vaccine response is protective, but they are not available to the practicing clinician in the United States. As a result, the abnormal antibody response to Pneumovax23 is likely the largest contributor to the misdiagnosis of CVID and inappropriate use of immunoglobulin replacement.[2] The authors advise that responsiveness to Pneumovax23 should be interpreted with great caution when considering a diagnosis of CVID.

Classification

B-cell phenotypic classification schema originally stratified patients based on in vitro antibody production, but now they generally use surface marker phenotypes of peripheral B cells to group patients with CVID.[9] B-cell–based classification of patients with CVID using an *in vitro* functional antibody production assay generates the following 3 groups: no immunoglobulin production, immunoglobulin M (IgM) production only, or both normal IgM and IgG production. Because these outcomes are thought to just reflect either the absence or presence of class-switched and non–class-switched memory B cells in peripheral blood, similar classification of patients with CVID is achieved by a much simpler method using surface staining of peripheral B cells.[10] Two separate groups pioneered this approach using slightly different algorithms as outlined in **Fig. 1**.[10–12] These classification schemes were combined into the widely used EUROclass scheme with the following B-cell subsets measured: total B cells, IgD⁻ memory B cells, transitional B cells, and CD21^{lo} B cells.[13] Perturbations in these B-cell subclasses associate with disease features, such as splenomegaly and lymphoproliferation (see **Fig. 1**). Unfortunately, B-cell classification offers limited prognostic utility because of the low positive and negative predictive values. Further complicating the picture, a small fraction of patients with CVID change memory B-cell classification categories when monitored over a period time; however, the majority have stable B-cell phenotypes, at least in the short-term.[14]

Because patients with CVID often have varied clinical morbidities, they can be grouped based on the type of complications diagnosed. Using this approach, most patients in a large CVID cohort were grouped into a single mutually exclusive clinical category that seemed to be stable when followed longitudinally.[15] These original classifications were later refined to include only these 4 categories: no other disease-related complications, cytopenias, polyclonal lymphoproliferation, and unexplained persistent enteropathy.[16] The last 3 categories all associated with decreased survival, whereas a prolonged history of no CVID-associated comorbidity was a favorable prognostic indicator. Additional cohort studies confirmed that excess morbidity and mortality in patients with CVID comes from noninfectious complications; however, risk of poor outcomes varies quite significantly from cohort to cohort even when controlling for specific disease complications.[17–20]

Genetics

It is clear that genetic factors are largely responsible for the presentation and progression of CVID. The first line of evidence arises from a grouping of monogenic causes of CVID syndromes caused by biallelic deleterious mutations in *ICOS*, *TNFRSF13C* *CD19*, *CD20*, *CD21*, and *CD81*, and *TNFRSF13B*.[21–28] The second line of evidence arises from families in which there is a clear inheritance pattern of either CVID or IgA deficiency.[29] Third, several genetic polymorphisms inherited in a heterozygous fashion are seen with increased frequency in CVID populations compared with nonaffected controls. Heterozygous variants in TACI (**Box 1**) make up the bulk of these defects, but potentially contributing variants in BAFFR have been reported.[30] Finally, both genomic association and measurement of copy number variation have identified both genetic loci that cluster with disease and discreet genomic deletions and duplications that seem to be unique to patients with CVID when compared with controls.[31]

Several additional monogenic defects can result in a phenotypic expression that satisfies most criteria for a diagnosis of CVID. Examples include biallelic mutations in *LRBA* and *CD27*, as well as heterozygous variants in *CTLA4*, *PIK3CD*, *PLCG2*,

Table 1
Comparison of criteria for the diagnosis of CVID

		Conley et al,[1] 1999	Ameratunga et al,[3] 2013	ESID Registry,[4] 2014
Clinical features[a]		None defined	Clinical sequelae directly attributable to in vivo failure of the immune system (one or more criteria) • Recurrent, severe, or unusual infections • Poor response to antibiotics • Breakthrough bacterial infections despite prophylactic antibiotics • Infections despite immunization with the appropriate vaccine, for example, human papillomavirus disease • Bronchiectasis and/or chronic sinus disease • Inflammatory disorders or autoimmunity	One of the following: • Increased susceptibility to infection • Autoimmune manifestations • Granulomatous disease • Unexplained polyclonal lymphoproliferation • Affected family member with antibody deficiency
Antibody	IgG level	<2 SD of mean for age	<500 mg/dL for adults	<2 SD of mean for age (measured at least twice)
	IgA level	<2 SD of mean for age	<80 mg/dL for adults[b]	<2 SD of mean for age (measured at least twice)
	IgM level	<2 SD of mean for age	<40 mg/dL for adults[b]	<2 SD of mean for age
	Antibody response	Either: • Poor antibody response to vaccines • Absent isohemagglutinins	• Impaired vaccine responses compared with age-matched controls[b] • Transient responses to vaccines compared with age-matched controls[b] • Absent isohemagglutinins	Either: • Poor antibody response to vaccines • Absent isohemagglutinins
	B cells	—	• Presence of B cells but reduced memory B cell subsets and/or increased CD21[lo] subsets by flow cytometry[b]	Or low switched memory B cells (<70% of age-related normal value)
	Other	—	• IgG3 <20 mg/dL[b] • Serologic support for autoimmunity[b] • Sequence variations of genes predisposing to CVID[b]	—

Age	Age >2 y	Age >4 y	Age ≥4 y
T cells	—	—	NOT any of the following: • CD4 numbers per microliter: 2–6 y <00, 6–12 y <250, >12 y <200 • % Naive CD4: 2–6 y <25%, 6–16 y <20%, >16 y <10% • T-cell proliferation absent
Pathologic findings	—	*Histologic markers of CVID*[c] • Lymphoid interstitial pneumonitis • Granulomatous disorder • Nodular regenerative hyperplasia of the liver • Nodular lymphoid hyperplasia of the gut • Absence of plasma cells on gut biopsy	—

Supportive criteria are in italics. All other criteria are mandatory.
[a] All 3 systems indicate that secondary causes of hypogammaglobulinemia must be ruled out for a diagnosis of CVID.
[b] Supportive laboratory criteria. Three or more are required to fulfill the category.
[c] Not required for diagnosis but supportive.
Data from Refs.[1,3,4]

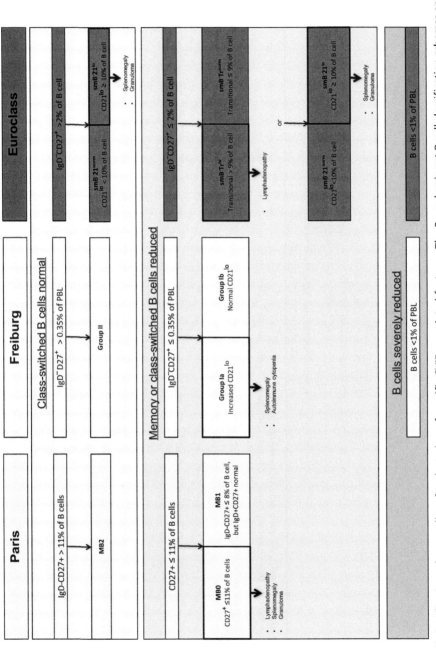

Fig. 1. B-cell classification schemas allow for clustering of specific CVID-associated features. The 3 predominant B-cell classification schemas are represented. All 3 categorize patients based on normal or low numbers of memory B-cell subsets; additionally, the Freiburg and Euroclass systems subcategorize patients based on numbers of transitional B cells and CD21^{lo} B cells. Class-switched B cell = CD19$^+$ CD27$^+$ IgD$^-$; transitional B cell = CD19$^+$ sIgM^{hi}CD38hi; CD21^{lo} = CD19$^+$ CD38^{lo}CD21^{lo}; PBL, peripheral blood lymphocyte; sm, switched memory; Tr, transitional. (*Data from* Refs. [10–13])

Box 1
The Role of TACI variants in CVID

Mutations in the gene *TNFRSF13B*, or TACI, are the most frequently identified genetic lesions that potentially play a role in the development of CVID. Variations in *TNFRSF13B* were initially identified in 2 separate cohorts of patients with CVID, and it seemed that the variants were not detected in healthy controls or unaffected family members.[27,28] Evaluation of larger populations showed that several variations could be found in both healthy controls and healthy first-degree relatives of patients with CVID; however, the most prevalent variation, C104R, was consistently found to increase the odds ratio of having CVID, even in the heterozygous state.[120,121] Further investigations confirmed the additional observation that biallelic pathogenic variations are not found in healthy control populations, particularly with regard to the common C104R variant and other variants highly likely to be deleterious to the formed protein.[122,123] These findings confirm that at least some *TNFRSF13B* genetic variations contribute to the onset of CVID in susceptible patients.

Investigation into the mechanism by which *TNFRSF13B* defects contribute to CVID have been hampered by the difficulty in distinguishing the effect of the TACI defect from underlying immune dysregulation; however, more recent studies have been able to attribute characteristic abnormalities in the immune system to the defective TACI protein. Initial studies demonstrated defective binding of both BAFF and A proliferation-inducing ligand (APRIL) to the C104R allele, and they also showed impaired downstream effects of stimulation using these 2 B-cell activators.[27,28] Subsequently, these observations were extended to healthy individuals that carried one of the defective alleles, adding the observation that TACI levels were reduced in all *TNFRSF13B* heterozygotes independent of CVID status.[124] Most recently, both central B-cell tolerance and B-cell activation were shown to be abnormal in individuals with either single or biallelic deleterious *TNFRSF13B* mutations independent of CVID status.[64] In contrast, peripheral B-cell tolerance was intact in healthy individuals with a single pathogenic *TNFRSF13B* allele but not in patients with CVID with the same *TNFRSF13B* status. The summation of these findings suggests that even a single pathogenic *TNFRSF13B* variant results in an abnormal B-cell phenotype, but expression of disease depends on the loss of compensating forces.

Data from Refs.[27,28,64,120–124]

---

and likely several others.[32–37] Because several of these syndromes are thought to arise primarily from defective T-cell function, they are generally not classified within CVID even though these patients may fit the definition before their genetic diagnosis. It is anticipated that a substantial proportion of patients with a current diagnosis of CVID could similarly be removed from the diagnostic category based on improved understanding of the genetic underpinnings of such immune diseases.

Currently, there is no consensus to guide the genetic evaluation of patients with CVID. The compelling reasons for pursuing a genetic diagnosis include potential reclassification of a disease process, improved ability to anticipate complications, genetic counseling, and more specific therapy choices. Unfortunately, known monogenic causes of CVID make up the minority of CVID cases, and the genetics underlying most patients with CVID remain obscure.[38] Faced with an ever-growing list of genes that would need to be sequenced to rule out the minority causes of CVID, pursuing a genetic diagnosis in patients with CVID can be a daunting, costly, and impractical task. Next-generation sequencing methods, including exome sequencing and gene panels, hold the potential to decrease both the cost and the inconvenience of the pursuit. As a result, obtaining a comparative genomic hybridization array and broad panel sequencing in all patients with CVID, especially in patients with obvious CVID-associated clinical symptoms, may be a direction to pursue.[39]

Radiography

The diagnosis of CVID does not depend on radiographic findings, but imaging at the time of diagnosis can uncover concerning disease-associated complications. A chest computed tomography (CT) scan at the time of diagnosis can identify bronchiectasis, interstitial lung disease (ILD), and granulomatous lung disease, even in asymptomatic patients. Follow-up chest CT should be used judiciously because of the malignancy risk. MRI of the chest is a promising alternative, but its utility depends on having an expert radiologist in MRI lung imaging.[40] Abdominal ultrasound should be considered to accurately assess spleen size, intra-abdominal lymphadenopathy, and liver pathology.[41] Additional radiographic studies should be guided by presenting features.

EPIDEMIOLOGY

Because of the rarity of primary immunodeficiency in general, very large groups of patients with CVID have not been studied; however, there are several reports of CVID cohorts with substantial numbers of patients from which generalizations can be drawn (**Table 2**).[13,15,17,19,20,42–45] CVID occurs equally in males and females, although, among children, boys predominate. CVID age of onset is variable, but more recent studies suggest peaks in early childhood and around the third decade of life. Data on ethnicity and race are not adequate to draw conclusions. Several noninfectious complications are commonly reported, including splenomegaly, chronic gastrointestinal (GI) disease, bronchiectasis, chronic lung disease, autoimmune cytopenia, and other autoimmune, malignant, and granulomatous diseases. It is the presence of one or more of these noninfectious complications that in many ways defines CVID (see **Table 1**).

PATHOGENESIS
Cell Biology

Most patients with CVID have intrinsic B-cell defects. It has been known for some time that peripheral B cells from most patients with CVID produce subnormal amounts of IgG or IgM when subjected to B-cell receptor stimulation[9]; however, this finding may merely reflect the marked reduction of memory B cells in those patients with CVID.[10] Taking into account the variability in B-cell subsets contained in peripheral blood, several groups still have identified intrinsic B-cell abnormalities, including altered calcium signaling,[46,47] TLR7 and TLR9 signaling defects,[48] and impaired upregulation of activation markers.[49] Another recent study indicates that a subset of CVID may have defective early B-cell development in the bone marrow.[50] These defects are variably present in patients with CVID, underlying the significant heterogeneity of this disease population.

Several studies suggest a primary role for T-cell abnormalities in the progression of CVID; however, recent efforts to reclassify patients with primary T-cell abnormalities have generated some confusion as to what degree T-cell defects contribute to CVID. Several studies have identified decreases in the number of naive CD4 cells in the peripheral blood of some patients with CVID,[51–54] and there is some evidence suggesting defective generation of T-cell precursors in the bone marrow.[55] Likewise, patients with CVID have decreased numbers of regulatory T cells (Treg) in the peripheral blood.[56–58] Additional T-cell defects identified in subsets of patients with CVID include defective upregulation of CD40L,[59,60] increased apoptosis,[61,62] and defective cytokine release in response to stimulatory molecules.[62,63] It is possible that these abnormalities were identified in CVID groups containing patients that would no longer be

Table 2
Epidemiology of recent CVID cohorts

Study	Population	No. Patients	Sex Distribution Female	Bronchiectasis/Chronic Lung Disease	Autoimmunity	GI Disease (Include Liver)	Lymphoproliferation	Granuloma	Malignancy
Quinti et al,[42] 2007	Italy	224	50%	29%	26%	28% Gastritis, 22% chronic diarrhea	26.4% Splenomegaly	—	6% Lymphoma
Chapel et al,[15] 2008	Mixed Europe	424	42%	4%–52%	7% ITP; 4% AHA; 5% vitiligo; 9% pernicious anemia	3%–15%	3% to 66% Splenomegaly	2–10%	6%
Resnick et al,[17] 2012	New York, United States	473	56%	29% CLD; 11% bronchiectasis	29%	15% Inflammatory; 6% malabsorption; 9% liver	—	10%	8% Lymphoma; 7% other
Wehr et al,[13] 2008	Mixed Europe	303	56%	—	20% General; 20% cytopenia	—	40.5% Splenomegaly; 26% lymphadenopathy	12%	—
Oksenhendler et al,[43] 2008	France	252	56%	37% Bronchiectasis	18% Cytopenia	23% Chronic diarrhea	38% Splenomegaly	14%	6% Lymphoma
Aghamohammadi et al,[20] 2014	Iran	173[a]	47%	—	15% Cytopenia	10% Enteropathy	37% Polyclonal lymphocytic infiltration	—	11%
Lin et al,[44] 2015	China	40	25%	—	15% General	—	—	—	—
Ramírez-Vargas et al,[45] 2014	Mexico	43	47%	51% Bronchiectasis	23% General	44% Noninfectious diarrhea	9% Splenomegaly; lymphadenopathy 67%	—	2%
Gathmann et al,[19] 2014	Mixed Europe	2212	51%[b]	0%–66%	0%–50%	0%–21% Enteropathy	0%–62% Splenomegaly	0–18%	0%–13% Lymphoma

Abbreviations: AHA, autoimmune hemolytic anemia; CLD, chronic lung disease; ITP, idiopathic thrombocytopenic purpura.
[a] 61.2% consanguineous parents.
[b] 33% in those aged 4 to 11 year old; 36% younger than 18 years old.
Data from Refs.[13,15,17,19,20,42–45]

considered as CVID; however, at least one recent study using strict diagnostic criteria and studying patients with known *TNFRSF13B* mutations identified expansions of T follicular helper cells and confirmed decreased Treg numbers in patients with CVID.[64] Together, these studies indicate that intrinsic T-cell defects are likely contributors to at least a portion of patients with CVID.

Defects in the dendritic cell (DC) compartment are also present within selected patients with CVID. Both plasmacytoid and myeloid DCs are present in decreased number in the peripheral blood of patients with CVID.[65,66] Whether these remaining cells have altered function remains controversial. The reason for the decrease in DC number is not known. There is no quantitative abnormality of DC precursors in bone marrow, and they do not seem to accumulate in tissues.[67]

Role of Chronic Immune Activation

Recent lines of investigation have identified evidence of chronic immune system activation in CVID. Evidence of chronic activation has been noted on T cells,[68,69] invariably natural killer T cells (iNKT),[68] and monocytes.[70] Serum evidence of chronic immune activation includes elevated sCD14 levels in blood of patients with CVID.[68,70] The cause of this chronic immune activation phenotype is unknown, but the finding of exhausted bacteria-specific T cells and detectable lipopolysaccharide levels in the plasma of patients with CVID not receiving adequate immunoglobulin replacement suggests that bacterial translocation from the GI tract may play a role.[69]

Intravenous immunoglobulin (IVIG) treatment, even at replacement doses, may partially alleviate the chronic inflammatory state; but more study needs to be performed. Immunoglobulin G, both in vivo and in vitro, has been shown to transiently decrease numbers of inflammatory monocytes,[71] increase numbers of Treg,[72] increase interferon-γ production by iNKT cells,[73] and correct some of the DC phenotypic abnormalities found in patients with CVID.[74] Despite these immediate antiinflammatory changes, T-cell exhaustion and even the inflammatory monocyte phenotype seem to persist in the long-term while patients receive immunoglobulin replacement. In the absence of evidence of long-lasting resolution of chronic immune activation, it is unlikely that IVIG alone is adequate treatment; however, it does suggest that the benefit of immunoglobulin replacement in CVID extends beyond infection prevention and includes some beneficial antiinflammatory effects.[74–76]

MANAGEMENT
Prognosis

The diagnosis of CVID carries a significantly increased mortality risk; however, the risk seems to be entirely contained within a subset of patients. The increased mortality risk was initially attributed to noninfectious complications in a large retrospective analysis of a European CVID registry.[15] Confirming that finding, a large single-center study identified an 11-times higher risk of death among patients with CVID with noninfectious complications compared with patients with CVID with only infectious complications.[17] Earlier studies were unable to assign the mortality risk to a particular subgroup; however, mortality risk was previously reported as being higher in the past than it is today.[77] As a group, these studies suggest that, although infection-related mortality has decreased, the risk of death from noninfectious complications remains quite significant.

The subset of patients with noninfectious complications faces significant risk of early mortality. Overall, studies report deaths in patients with malignancy, chronic lung disease, infection, and liver disease.[15,42,77] More recent studies show that risk of early death is experienced exclusively in patients with noninfectious CVID morbidities.[15,17] As a result, it is important to identify those patients with CVID with severe noninfectious complications and institute therapy where possible.

Clinical Monitoring

Patients with CVID suffer from diverse complications; as a result, clinical monitoring guidelines have not reached a universal consensus. In the absence of clear guidelines for clinical monitoring, the authors recommend the following: initial evaluation should seek to determine the presence of CVID-associated comorbidity, such as lymphoproliferative disease, lung disease, liver disease, and autoimmunity (**Table 3**). Ongoing monitoring includes the following: verifying serum IgG levels to ensure patients are receiving adequate immunoglobulin replacement, monitoring for the presence or onset of CVID-associated complications not initially present at the time of diagnosis, and monitoring for deterioration of comorbidities diagnosed at presentation. Intervals in which these screening activities should occur is not clear, but patients may require being seen and evaluated multiple times yearly. These frequent monitoring intervals particularly apply to patients receiving replacement IgG at home or at off-site locations who would otherwise be seen less frequently.

Treatment Approach

Effective treatment of CVID depends on adequate treatment of both infectious and noninfectious medical issues. IgG replacement is generally effective in preventing further infections, although, for patients who have bronchiectasis, aggressive pulmonary physiotherapy should also be implemented. Antibiotic prophylaxis is frequently used in patients with persistent infections; however, this practice is controversial. Both antifungal and antiviral prophylaxis generally are not required, and patients with recurrent fungal or severe viral infections should be evaluated for a combined immunodeficiency syndrome. Treatment of noninfectious complications requires specific management approaches tailored to the specific problem. Medications can include immunosuppressives and even cytotoxic therapies. There is limited experience with organ transplantation; similarly, bone marrow transplantation has been reported retrospectively and in few patients.[78,79]

Table 3	
Suggested baseline clinical screening for patients with CVID	
Specific Complication	**Baseline Screening Recommendation**
Liver disease	AST, ALT, GGT, Alk phos Abdominal ultrasound with Doppler
Intestinal disease	Upper/lower endoscopy
Lung disease	CT chest Pulmonary function testing Lung diffusion capacity
Cytopenia	CBC Lymphocyte phenotype
Malignancy	CBC, LDH
Lymphoproliferation	Abdominal ultrasound

Abbreviations: Alk phos, alkaline phosphatase; ALT, alanine transaminase; AST, aspartate transaminase; CBC, complete blood count; GGT, gamma-glutamyl transpeptidase; LDH, lactate dehydrogenase.

Specific Complications

Diseases of the gastrointestinal tract and liver

GI inflammatory disease is common in CVID. Manifestations can be varied and include chronic enteropathy, inflammatory bowel disease, gastritis, and pernicious anemia; however, chronic enteropathy is the most common complication. Typical macroscopic findings of CVID-associated enteropathy include nodular lymphoid hyperplasia and nonspecific inflammation. Microscopic findings reveal an absence of plasma cells, intraepithelial infiltration of lymphocytes, and hyperplastic lymphoid follicles.[80] Other findings can include villous blunting and crypt apoptosis. The cause of CVID enteropathy is not known. Occasionally, infectious organisms, such as *Giardia lamblia, Cryptosporidium parvum, cytomegalovirus, Salmonella* species, and *Campylobacter jejuni*, are isolated; but frequently no infectious organism is found.[81] Enteric viruses are more likely to be identified in the GI tract of patients with CVID; however, most of these viruses clear within 3 months.[82] In one cohort recently described, some adult patients with CVID with chronic enteropathy had evidence of chronic norovirus infection that in 2 patients resolved with ribavirin therapy.[83] For patients without a clear infectious cause, improvement with anti–tumor necrosis factor (TNF) therapy has been reported.[84]

Liver disease in CVID is varied, including idiopathic abnormalities of the portal circulation, primary biliary cirrhosis, hepatitis, and nodular regenerative hyperplasia (NRH).[81] NRH is the most common severe liver disease, being confirmed in up to 5% of patients with CVID.[85] NRH is frequently associated with lymphocytic infiltrates, stable fibrosis, and inflammatory enteropathy.[85,86] Granulomas can also be seen on biopsy. The natural history of NRH is not clear because no screening study has been performed to assess the true prevalence of NRH in the CVID population. As portal circulation abnormalities and elevated liver enzymes are commonly seen in CVID,[41,85] it is possible that NRH is more common than previously thought. In patients with CVID where the symptoms are severe enough to necessitate biopsy, the clinical course is generally poor with most patients developing portal hypertension and cirrhosis.

Liver disease can be an ominous comorbidity in CVID; as a result, it should be managed aggressively. NRH has the capacity for gradual or even rapid progression to hepatitis and portal hypertension resulting in splenomegaly, ascites, varices, and even liver synthetic dysfunction.[85] If prolonged liver enzyme abnormalities are identified or there is other evidence of liver dysfunction, biopsy should be considered. If NRH is identified, the amount of inflammatory infiltrate needs to be assessed; if present, immunosuppressive treatment should be considered. There is no apparent link between length of IVIG usage and NRH development, and replacement immunoglobulin therapy should not be discontinued.[87] Liver transplantation likely should not be performed in light of the high likelihood of graft rejection.[88]

Pulmonary disease

Lung disease in patients with CVID is generally divided between disease of the airways and interstitial lung disease. Airway disease includes infection, obstructive disease, and bronchiectasis. Bronchiectasis is attributable to a history of underlying pulmonary infection but also can be seen in patients with no history of pulmonary infection.[89] Interstitial lung diseases include granuloma, organizing pneumonia, and lymphoid infiltrative disease with or without a follicular arrangement.[90,91] Combined infiltrative lymphocytic and granulomatous lung disease is referred to as granulomatous lymphocytic interstitial lymphocytic disease (GLILD). GLILD occurs less frequently than other forms of chronic lung disease, and it carries a significantly increased mortality risk both because of progression and because of frequent association with additional CVID-related morbidity.[92,93] As a category, pulmonary disease is very common in CVID; in one recent study, CT screening identified bronchiectasis in 64% of patients and evidence of ILD in 72% of patients.[89]

Treatment of pulmonary disease is targeted at the underlying problem. Bronchiectasis is not reversed by initiation of replacement immunoglobulin therapy; however, adequate immunoglobulin replacement is essential to prevent bacterial reinfection and disease progression.[94] Routine pulmonary physiotherapy to enhance mucus clearance should be continued lifelong. Effective treatment of interstitial lung disease has been reported with the use of rituximab and azathioprine, although the duration of response is not clear.[91,95] There are limited data reporting the experience with other immunosuppressive medications.[96] To some extent the histopathology may be helpful in choosing therapy. In those with exclusive T-cell infiltration, corticosteroids and other T-cell targeted therapies may attenuate disease. In those with significant B-cell infiltration and follicle formation, steroids may be less effective and require alternative approaches.

Anemia and thrombocytopenia

Blood cell autoimmunity affecting both platelets and red blood cells, either independently or simultaneously, is the most frequent autoimmune complication in CVID.[77] Autoimmune neutropenia can also occur albeit with less frequency. Between 10% and 20% of patients have autoimmune cytopenia; among these patients, cytopenia is frequently the first clue to the diagnosis of CVID.[97] Cytopenia is frequently associated with splenomegaly, which is likely the cause of cytopenia in some, but it also can exist in the absence of splenomegaly.[13] Autoimmune cytopenia is diagnosed the same way in patients with CVID as in nonimmunodeficient patients.

There are limited data on the proper treatment of autoimmune cytopenia in CVID, partially because of the small number of patients and also because most patients present with idiopathic thrombocytopenic purpura (ITP) before being diagnosed with CVID. As a result, autoimmune cytopenia treatment is similar to treatment of patients without CVID; but there should be consideration of the fact that the patients already have increased infection susceptibility. Initiation of immunoglobulin replacement does not seem to resolve ITP; however, it is important to ensure adequate replacement because ITP treatments are potentially immunosuppressive.[98] Initial treatment of ITP consists of prolonged oral corticosteroid treatment. If corticosteroids are thought to be ineffective, high-dose IVIG can be trialed, although many patients will remain refractory.[99,100] If the condition remains refractory, rituximab can be considered as a second-line therapy.[100] Rituximab treatment at standard dosing in one retrospective study achieved a durable response in 50% of patients with refractory cytopenia.[99] B-cell phenotyping should be performed before the initiation of rituximab. Immunomodulators and splenectomy are reserved as a last resort in patients who have failed all other therapies, and they are generally disfavored because of risk of subsequent infection.[100] Treatment of autoimmune hemolytic anemia (AIHA) is identical to ITP; although, the response to high-dose IVIG is lower in AIHA and relapse should be anticipated.[98]

Granuloma

Granulomas arise in a minority of individuals with CVID. Granuloma in a single location is frequently accompanied by additional granulomas in other body sites.[93,101] The lung is the most commonly affected organ.[101] Additional locations include spleen, lymph nodes, liver, bowel, bone marrow, skin, brain, parotid, retina, and kidney.[101,102]

Granulomas can vary in size,[102] and they can appear within and outside of lymphoid follicles.[103] They are most frequently non-necrotizing.[104] The presence of granuloma in CVID significantly increases the likelihood of associated autoimmunity and spleno-megaly.[101,105] Combined with the fact that the cause of granuloma is almost univer-sally not traceable to an infectious microorganism, the association with other autoimmunity suggests that granuloma formation is linked to widespread immune dysregulation.

Effective treatment of granuloma has not been established. Corticosteroid therapy is frequently used and in one retrospective study was at least partially effective in a fraction of patients with granuloma.[101] IVIG even at high doses does not induce remis-sion. Infliximab treatment resulted in clinical improvement in 5 patients with CVID whose granulomatous disease was refractory to other immunosuppressive therapy, including steroids.[106] Additional case reports indicate a favorable responses to TNF-blocking agents in CVID-associated granuloma.[104,107,108]

Malignancy

Malignancy is an occasional event in CVID, and it is a major cause of early mortality in adult CVID cohorts. Upwards of 20% of adult patients with CVID develop some form of cancer.[109] The most common form is lymphoma, but nonhematopoietic cancers have been reported. Early studies indicated greater than a 33-times increased risk of either lymphoma or gastric cancer in patients with CVID[110]; however, more recent studies have identified only a modestly increased risk of lymphoma.[111]

Arthritis

Joint involvement includes both infectious and noninfectious processes. Infection with *Mycoplasma* and *Ureaplasma* species can rarely cause low-grade chronic joint inflam-mation if left untreated.[112] Noninfectious inflammation of the joints, including both large and small joints, is reported to resolve with initiation of IVIG; however, cases of persistent and destructive arthritis have been reported.[113,114] In general, treatment of inflammatory arthritis in CVID is the same as when CVID is not present.[115,116]

Infection

The risk of severe infection in CVID is largely ameliorated by adequate immunoglobulin replacement therapy, but less severe infections can persist. For patients on replacement immunoglobulin, ongoing infections include mainly upper- and lower-respiratory tract infection with either bacteria or respiratory viruses,[117] with sinus infec-tion being far more common than pneumonia.[18] Some studies have suggested that achieving increased IgG trough levels can decrease the rate of these residual infections in CVID,[118,119] although others have not recognized an advantage of increasing IgG trough levels greater than 600 mg/dL. These data indicate that, for most patients with CVID, the infection susceptibility remains limited to the humoral immune compartment and replacement of IgG effectively compensates for the humoral immune deficiency.

CONCLUDING REMARKS

Over the past 60 years, CVID has emerged as the predominant class of primary anti-body deficiencies. During this time period, important variation in both clinical features and underlying pathology have been identified. In fact, many patients with CVID have little in common other than meeting minimal diagnostic criteria. Nonetheless, grouping patients with antibody deficiency into this diagnostic category has allowed for the dif-ferentiation of multiple important endotypes, the study of which will likely reveal key mechanisms underlying the disease features currently associated with CVID.

Combining modern genetic approaches and an improved understanding of immunobiology, researchers are likely to continue to clarify the subtypes of CVID, possibly to the point when CVID is no longer a useful disease classification.

While waiting for research advancements to be translated into treatment, clinicians who care for these patients must remain diligent in providing comprehensive screening, monitoring, and treatment catered specifically to this population. Clinical testing thresholds are different from the healthy population, and clinicians managing patients with CVID must calibrate these thresholds based on the array of morbidities that arise in these patients. Phenotypic classification schemes can help physicians anticipate some of the types of problems they may encounter; however, none of the systems are perfect. For treatment, IgG replacement is essential; but the specter of noninfectious CVID-related morbidity poses the greatest threat to the health of patients with CVID. As a result, the combination of a high index of suspicion and clinical acumen still represents the best hope in avoiding negative outcomes in this complex disease category.

REFERENCES

1. Conley ME, Notarangelo LD, Etzioni A. Diagnostic criteria for primary immunodeficiencies. Representing PAGID (Pan-American Group for Immunodeficiency) and ESID (European Society for Immunodeficiencies). Clin Immunol 1999;93(3): 190–7.
2. Gelfand EW, Ochs HD, Shearer WT. Controversies in IgG replacement therapy in patients with antibody deficiency diseases. J Allergy Clin Immunol 2013; 131(4):1001–5.
3. Ameratunga R, Woon ST, Gillis D, et al. New diagnostic criteria for common variable immune deficiency (CVID), which may assist with decisions to treat with intravenous or subcutaneous immunoglobulin. Clin Exp Immunol 2013; 174(2):203–11.
4. European Society for Immunodeficiencies Registry Working Party. Available at: http://esid.org/Working-Parties/Registry/Diagnosis-criteria. Accessed August 10, 2015.
5. Jaffe EF, Lejtenyi MC, Noya FJ, et al. Secondary hypogammaglobulinemia. Immunol Allergy Clin N Am 2001;21(1):141–63.
6. da Silva SP, Resnick E, Lucas M, et al. Lymphoid proliferations of indeterminate malignant potential arising in adults with common variable immunodeficiency disorders: unusual case studies and immunohistological review in the light of possible causative events. J Clin Immunol 2011;31(5):784–91.
7. Daly TM, Pickering JW, Zhang X, et al. Multilaboratory assessment of threshold versus fold-change algorithms for minimizing analytical variability in multiplexed pneumococcal IgG measurements. Clin Vaccin Immunol 2014;21(7):982–8.
8. Balloch A, Licciardi PV, Tang MLK. Serotype-specific anti-pneumococcal IgG and immune competence: critical differences in interpretation criteria when different methods are used. J Clin Immunol 2013;33(2):335–41.
9. Bryant A, Calver NC, Toubi E, et al. Classification of patients with common variable immunodeficiency by B cell secretion of IgM and IgG in response to anti-IgM and interleukin-2. Clin Immunol Immunopathol 1990;56(2):239–48.
10. Warnatz K, Denz A, Dräger R, et al. Severe deficiency of switched memory B cells (CD27(+)IgM(−)IgD(−)) in subgroups of patients with common variable immunodeficiency: a new approach to classify a heterogeneous disease. Blood 2002;99(5):1544–51.

11. Piqueras B, Lavenu-Bombled C, Galicier L, et al. Common variable immunodeficiency patient classification based on impaired B cell memory differentiation correlates with clinical aspects. J Clin Immunol 2003;23(5):385–400.
12. Warnatz K, Wehr C, Dräger R, et al. Expansion of CD19(hi)CD21(lo/neg) B cells in common variable immunodeficiency (CVID) patients with autoimmune cytopenia. Immunobiology 2002;206(5):502–13.
13. Wehr C, Kivioja T, Schmitt C, et al. The EUROclass trial: defining subgroups in common variable immunodeficiency. Blood 2008;111(1):77–85.
14. Koopmans W, Woon ST, Zeng ISL, et al. Variability of memory B cell markers in a cohort of common variable immune deficiency patients over 6 months. Scand J Immunol 2013;77(6):470–5.
15. Chapel H, Lucas M, Lee M, et al. Common variable immunodeficiency disorders: division into distinct clinical phenotypes. Blood 2008;112(2):277–86.
16. Chapel H, Lucas M, Patel S, et al. Confirmation and improvement of criteria for clinical phenotyping in common variable immunodeficiency disorders in replicate cohorts. J Allergy Clin Immunol 2012;130(5):1197–8.e9.
17. Resnick ES, Moshier EL, Godbold JH, et al. Morbidity and mortality in common variable immune deficiency over 4 decades. Blood 2012;119(7):1650–7.
18. Quinti I, Soresina A, Guerra A, et al. Effectiveness of immunoglobulin replacement therapy on clinical outcome in patients with primary antibody deficiencies: results from a multicenter prospective cohort study. J Clin Immunol 2011;31(3): 315–22.
19. Gathmann B, Mahlaoui N, CEREDIH, et al. Clinical picture and treatment of 2212 patients with common variable immunodeficiency. J Allergy Clin Immunol 2014; 134(1):116–26.
20. Aghamohammadi A, Abolhassani H, Latif A, et al. Long-term evaluation of a historical cohort of Iranian common variable immunodeficiency patients. Exp Rev Clin Immunol 2014;10(10):1405–17.
21. Grimbacher B, Hutloff A, Schlesier M, et al. Homozygous loss of ICOS is associated with adult-onset common variable immunodeficiency. Nat Immunol 2003; 4(3):261–8.
22. Warnatz K, Salzer U, Rizzi M, et al. B-cell activating factor receptor deficiency is associated with an adult-onset antibody deficiency syndrome in humans. Proc Natl Acad Sci U S A 2009;106(33):13945–50.
23. van Zelm MC, Reisli I, van der Burg M, et al. An antibody-deficiency syndrome due to mutations in the CD19 gene. N Engl J Med 2006;354(18):1901–12.
24. Kuijpers TW, Bende RJ, Baars PA, et al. CD20 deficiency in humans results in impaired T cell-independent antibody responses. J Clin Invest 2010;120(1):214–22.
25. Thiel J, Kimmig L, Salzer U, et al. Genetic CD21 deficiency is associated with hypogammaglobulinemia. J Allergy Clin Immunol 2012;129(3):801–10.e6.
26. van Zelm MC, Smet J, Adams B, et al. CD81 gene defect in humans disrupts CD19 complex formation and leads to antibody deficiency. J Clin Invest 2010; 120(4):1265–74.
27. Castigli E, Wilson SA, Garibyan L, et al. TACI is mutant in common variable immunodeficiency and IgA deficiency. Nat Genet 2005;37(8):829–34.
28. Salzer U, Chapel HM, Webster ADB, et al. Mutations in TNFRSF13B encoding TACI are associated with common variable immunodeficiency in humans. Nat Genet 2005;37(8):820–8.
29. Vorechovsky I, Zetterquist H, Paganelli R, et al. Family and linkage study of selective IgA deficiency and common variable immunodeficiency. Clin Immunol Immunopathol 1995;77(2):185–92.

30. Pieper K, Rizzi M, Speletas M, et al. A common single nucleotide polymorphism impairs B-cell activating factor receptor's multimerization, contributing to common variable immunodeficiency. J Allergy Clin Immunol 2014;133(4):1222–5.
31. Orange JS, Glessner JT, Resnick E, et al. Genome-wide association identifies diverse causes of common variable immunodeficiency. J Allergy Clin Immunol 2011;127(6):1360–7.e6.
32. Lopez-Herrera G, Tampella G, Pan-Hammarström Q, et al. Deleterious mutations in LRBA are associated with a syndrome of immune deficiency and autoimmunity. Am J Hum Genet 2012;90(6):986–1001.
33. van Montfrans JM, Hoepelman AIM, Otto S, et al. CD27 deficiency is associated with combined immunodeficiency and persistent symptomatic EBV viremia. J Allergy Clin Immunol 2012;129(3):787–93.e6.
34. Kuehn HS, Ouyang W, Lo B, et al. Immune dysregulation in human subjects with heterozygous germline mutations in CTLA4. Science 2014;345(6204):1623–7.
35. Schubert D, Bode C, Kenefeck R, et al. Autosomal dominant immune dysregulation syndrome in humans with CTLA4 mutations. Nat Med 2014;20(12):1410–6.
36. Lucas CL, Kuehn HS, Zhao F, et al. Dominant-activating germline mutations in the gene encoding the PI(3)K catalytic subunit p110δ result in T cell senescence and human immunodeficiency. Nat Immunol 2013;15(1):88–97.
37. Ombrello MJ, Remmers EF, Sun G, et al. Cold urticaria, immunodeficiency, and autoimmunity related to PLCG2 deletions. N Engl J Med 2012;366(4):330–8.
38. Ochs HD. Common variable immunodeficiency (CVID): new genetic insight and unanswered questions. Clin Exp Immunol 2014;178(Suppl 1):5–6.
39. Seppänen M, Aghamohammadi A, Rezaei N. Is there a need to redefine the diagnostic criteria for common variable immunodeficiency? Exp Rev Clin Immunol 2014;10(1):1–5.
40. Montella S, Maglione M, Bruzzese D, et al. Magnetic resonance imaging is an accurate and reliable method to evaluate non-cystic fibrosis paediatric lung disease. Respirology 2012;17(1):87–91.
41. Pulvirenti F, Pentassuglio I, Milito C, et al. Idiopathic non cirrhotic portal hypertension and splenoportal axis abnormalities in patients with severe primary antibody deficiencies. J Immunol Res 2014;2014:672458.
42. Quinti I, Soresina A, Spadaro G, et al. Long-term follow-up and outcome of a large cohort of patients with common variable immunodeficiency. J Clin Immunol 2007;27(3):308–16.
43. Oksenhendler E, Gérard L, Fieschi C, et al. Infections in 252 patients with common variable immunodeficiency. Clin Infect Dis 2008;46(10):1547–54.
44. Lin L-J, Wang Y-C, Liu X-M. Clinical and immunological features of common variable immunodeficiency in China. Chin Med J 2015;128(3):310–5.
45. Ramírez-Vargas N, Arablin-Oropeza SE, Mojica-Martínez D, et al. Clinical and immunological features of common variable immunodeficiency in Mexican patients. Allergol Immunopathol (Madr) 2014;42(3):235–40.
46. van de Ven AAJM, Compeer EB, Bloem AC, et al. Defective calcium signaling and disrupted CD20-B-cell receptor dissociation in patients with common variable immunodeficiency disorders. J Allergy Clin Immunol 2012;129(3):755–61.e7.
47. Foerster C, Voelxen N, Rakhmanov M, et al. B cell receptor-mediated calcium signaling is impaired in B lymphocytes of type Ia patients with common variable immunodeficiency. J Immunol 2010;184(12):7305–13.
48. Yu JE, Knight AK, Radigan L, et al. Toll-like receptor 7 and 9 defects in common variable immunodeficiency. J Allergy Clin Immunol 2009;124(2):349–56, 356.e1–3.

49. Groth C, Drager R, Warnatz K, et al. Impaired up-regulation of CD70 and CD86 in naive (CD27-) B cells from patients with common variable immunodeficiency (CVID). Clin Exp Immunol 2002;129(1):133–9.

50. Anzilotti C, Kienzler A-K, Lopez-Granados E, et al. Key stages of bone marrow B-cell maturation are defective in patients with common variable immunodeficiency disorders. J Allergy Clin Immunol 2015.

51. Guazzi V, Aiuti F, Mezzaroma I, et al. Assessment of thymic output in common variable immunodeficiency patients by evaluation of T cell receptor excision circles. Clin Exp Immunol 2002;129(2):346–53.

52. Isgrò A, Marziali M, Mezzaroma I, et al. Bone marrow clonogenic capability, cytokine production, and thymic output in patients with common variable immunodeficiency. J Immunol 2005;174(8):5074–81.

53. Oraei M, Aghamohammadi A, Rezaei N, et al. Naive CD4+ T cells and recent thymic emigrants in common variable immunodeficiency. J Investig Allergol Clin Immunol 2012;22(3):160–7.

54. Serana F, Airo P, Chiarini M, et al. Thymic and bone marrow output in patients with common variable immunodeficiency. J Clin Immunol 2011;31(4):540–9.

55. Ochtrop MLG, Goldacker S, May AM, et al. T and B lymphocyte abnormalities in bone marrow biopsies of common variable immunodeficiency. Blood 2011; 118(2):309–18.

56. Melo KM, Carvalho KI, Bruno FR, et al. A decreased frequency of regulatory T cells in patients with common variable immunodeficiency. PLoS ONE 2009;4(7): e6269.

57. Horn J, Manguiat A, Berglund LJ, et al. Decrease in phenotypic regulatory T cells in subsets of patients with common variable immunodeficiency. Clin Exp Immunol 2009;156(3):446–54.

58. Arandi N, Mirshafiey A, Jeddi-Tehrani M, et al. Evaluation of CD4+CD25+FOXP3+ regulatory T cells function in patients with common variable immunodeficiency. Cell Immunol 2013;281(2):129–33.

59. Farrington M, Grosmaire LS, Nonoyama S, et al. CD40 ligand expression is defective in a subset of patients with common variable immunodeficiency. Proc Natl Acad Sci U S A 1994;91(3):1099–103.

60. Oliva A, Scala E, Quinti I, et al. IL-10 production and CD40L expression in patients with common variable immunodeficiency. Scand J Immunol 1997;46(1):86–90.

61. Di Renzo M, Zhou Z, George I, et al. Enhanced apoptosis of T cells in common variable immunodeficiency (CVID): role of defective CD28 co-stimulation. Clin Exp Immunol 2000;120(3):503–11.

62. Giovannetti A, Pierdominici M, Mazzetta F, et al. Unravelling the complexity of T cell abnormalities in common variable immunodeficiency. J Immunol 2007; 178(6):3932–43.

63. Rezaei N, Aghamohammadi A, Nourizadeh M, et al. Cytokine production by activated T cells in common variable immunodeficiency. J Investig Allergol Clin Immunol 2010;20(3):244–51.

64. Romberg N, Chamberlain N, Saadoun D, et al. CVID-associated TACI mutations affect autoreactive B cell selection and activation. J Clin Invest 2013;123(10): 4283–93.

65. Viallard J-F, Camou F, André M, et al. Altered dendritic cell distribution in patients with common variable immunodeficiency. Arthritis Res Ther 2005;7(5):R1052–5.

66. Martinez-Pomar N, Raga S, Ferrer J, et al. Elevated serum interleukin (IL)-12p40 levels in common variable immunodeficiency disease and decreased peripheral

blood dendritic cells: analysis of IL-12p40 and interferon-gamma gene. Clin Exp Immunol 2006;144(2):233–8.

67. Taraldsrud E, Fevang B, Aukrust P, et al. Common variable immunodeficiency revisited: normal generation of naturally occurring dendritic cells that respond to Toll-like receptors 7 and 9. Clin Exp Immunol 2014;175(3):439–48.

68. Paquin-Proulx D, Santos BAN, Carvalho KI, et al. IVIG immune reconstitution treatment alleviates the state of persistent immune activation and suppressed CD4 T cell counts in CVID. PLoS One 2013;8(10):e75199.

69. Perreau M, Vigano S, Bellanger F, et al. Exhaustion of bacteria-specific CD4 T cells and microbial translocation in common variable immunodeficiency disorders. J Exp Med 2014;211(10):2033–45.

70. Barbosa RR, Silva SP, Silva SL, et al. Monocyte activation is a feature of common variable immunodeficiency irrespective of plasma lipopolysaccharide levels. Clin Exp Immunol 2012;169(3):263–72.

71. Siedlar M, Strach M, Bukowska-Strakova K, et al. Preparations of intravenous immunoglobulins diminish the number and proinflammatory response of CD14+CD16++ monocytes in common variable immunodeficiency (CVID) patients. Clin Immunol 2011;139(2):122–32.

72. Kasztalska K, Ciebiada M, Cebula-Obrzut B, et al. Intravenous immunoglobulin replacement therapy in the treatment of patients with common variable immunodeficiency disease: an open-label prospective study. Clin Drug Investig 2011; 31(5):299–307.

73. Gao Y, Workman S, Gadola S, et al. Common variable immunodeficiency is associated with a functional deficiency of invariant natural killer T cells. J Allergy Clin Immunol 2014;133(5):1420–8, 1428.e1.

74. Paquin-Proulx D, Sandberg JK. Persistent immune activation in CVID and the role of IVIG in its suppression. Front Immunol 2014;5:637.

75. Gelfand EW. Intravenous immune globulin in autoimmune and inflammatory diseases. N Engl J Med 2012;367(21):2015–25.

76. Kaveri SV, Maddur MS, Hegde P, et al. Intravenous immunoglobulins in immunodeficiencies: more than mere replacement therapy. Clin Exp Immunol 2011; 164(Suppl 2):2–5.

77. Cunningham-Rundles C, Bodian C. Common variable immunodeficiency: clinical and immunological features of 248 patients. Clin Immunol 1999;92(1): 34–48.

78. Rizzi M, Neumann C, Fielding AK, et al. Outcome of allogeneic stem cell transplantation in adults with common variable immunodeficiency. J Allergy Clin Immunol 2011;128(6):1371–4.e2.

79. Wehr C, Gennery AR, Lindemans C, et al. Multicenter experience in hematopoietic stem cell transplantation for serious complications of common variable immunodeficiency. J Allergy Clin Immunol 2015;135(4):988–97.

80. Malamut G, Verkarre V, Suarez F, et al. The enteropathy associated with common variable immunodeficiency: the delineated frontiers with celiac disease. Am J Gastroenterol 2010;105(10):2262–75.

81. Agarwal S, Mayer L. Diagnosis and treatment of gastrointestinal disorders in patients with primary immunodeficiency. Clin Gastroenterol Hepatol 2013;11(9): 1050–63.

82. van de Ven AAJM, Janssen WJM, Schulz LS, et al. Increased prevalence of gastrointestinal viruses and diminished secretory immunoglobulin A levels in antibody deficiencies. J Clin Immunol 2014;34(8):962–70.

83. Woodward JM, Gkrania-Klotsas E, Cordero-Ng AY, et al. The role of chronic norovirus infection in the enteropathy associated with common variable immunodeficiency. Am J Gastroenterol 2015;110(2):320–7.

84. Chua I, Standish R, Lear S, et al. Anti-tumour necrosis factor-alpha therapy for severe enteropathy in patients with common variable immunodeficiency (CVID). Clin Exp Immunol 2007;150(2):306–11.

85. Fuss IJ, Friend J, Yang Z, et al. Nodular regenerative hyperplasia in common variable immunodeficiency. J Clin Immunol 2013;33(4):748–58.

86. Daniels JA, Torbenson M, Vivekanandan P, et al. Hepatitis in common variable immunodeficiency. Hum Pathol 2009;40(4):484–8.

87. Ward C, Lucas M, Piris J, et al. Abnormal liver function in common variable immunodeficiency disorders due to nodular regenerative hyperplasia. Clin Exp Immunol 2008;153(3):331–7.

88. Murakawa Y, Miyagawa-Hayashino A, Ogura Y, et al. Liver transplantation for severe hepatitis in patients with common variable immunodeficiency. Pediatr Transplant 2012;16(6):E210–6.

89. Maarschalk-Ellerbroek LJ, de Jong PA, van Montfrans JM, et al. CT screening for pulmonary pathology in common variable immunodeficiency disorders and the correlation with clinical and immunological parameters. J Clin Immunol 2014; 34(6):642–54.

90. Hampson FA, Chandra A, Screaton NJ, et al. Respiratory disease in common variable immunodeficiency and other primary immunodeficiency disorders. Clin Radiol 2012;67(6):587–95.

91. Maglione PJ, Ko HM, Beasley MB, et al. Tertiary lymphoid neogenesis is a component of pulmonary lymphoid hyperplasia in patients with common variable immunodeficiency. J Allergy Clin Immunol 2014;133(2):535–42.

92. Bates CA, Ellison MC, Lynch DA, et al. Granulomatous- lymphocytic lung disease shortens survival in common variable immunodeficiency. J Allergy Clin Immunol 2004;114(2):415–21.

93. Bouvry D, Mouthon L, Brillet P-Y, et al. Granulomatosis-associated common variable immunodeficiency disorder: a case-control study versus sarcoidosis. Eur Respir J 2013;41(1):115–22.

94. Roifman CM, Levison H, Gelfand EW. High-dose versus low-dose intravenous immunoglobulin in hypogammaglobulinaemia and chronic lung disease. Lancet 1987;1(8541):1075–7.

95. Chase NM, Verbsky JW, Hintermeyer MK, et al. Use of combination chemotherapy for treatment of granulomatous and lymphocytic interstitial lung disease (GLILD) in patients with common variable immunodeficiency (CVID). J Clin Immunol 2012;33(1):30–9.

96. Prasse A, Kayser G, Warnatz K. Common variable immunodeficiency-associated granulomatous and interstitial lung disease. Curr Opin Pulm Med 2013;19(5):503–9.

97. Boileau J, Mouillot G, Gérard L, et al. Autoimmunity in common variable immunodeficiency: correlation with lymphocyte phenotype in the French DEFI study. J Autoimmun 2011;36(1):25–32.

98. Wang J, Cunningham-Rundles C. Treatment and outcome of autoimmune hematologic disease in common variable immunodeficiency (CVID). J Autoimmun 2005;25(1):57–62.

99. Gobert D, Bussel JB, Cunningham-Rundles C, et al. Efficacy and safety of rituximab in common variable immunodeficiency-associated immune cytopenias: a retrospective multicentre study on 33 patients. Br J Haematol 2011;155(4):498–508.

100. Cunningham-Rundles C. Hematologic complications of primary immune deficiencies. Blood Rev 2002;16(1):61–4.
101. Boursiquot J-N, Gérard L, Malphettes M, et al. Granulomatous disease in CVID: retrospective analysis of clinical characteristics and treatment efficacy in a cohort of 59 patients. J Clin Immunol 2013;33(1):84–95.
102. Ardeniz Ö, Cunningham-Rundles C. Granulomatous disease in common variable immunodeficiency. Clin Immunol 2009;133(2):198–207.
103. Unger S, Seidl M, Schmitt-Graeff A, et al. Ill-defined germinal centers and severely reduced plasma cells are histological hallmarks of lymphadenopathy in patients with common variable immunodeficiency. J Clin Immunol 2014; 34(6):615–26.
104. Hatab AZ, Ballas ZK. Caseating granulomatous disease in common variable immunodeficiency treated with infliximab. J Allergy Clin Immunol 2005;116(5):1161–2.
105. Mechanic LJ, Dikman S, Cunningham-Rundles C. Granulomatous disease in common variable immunodeficiency. Ann Intern Med 1997;127(8 Pt 1):613–7.
106. Franxman TJ, Howe LE, Baker JR. Infliximab for treatment of granulomatous disease in patients with common variable immunodeficiency. J Clin Immunol 2014; 34(7):820–7.
107. Lin JH, Liebhaber M, Roberts RL, et al. Etanercept treatment of cutaneous granulomas in common variable immunodeficiency. J Allergy Clin Immunol 2006; 117(4):878–82.
108. Thatayatikom A, Thatayatikom S, White AJ. Infliximab treatment for severe granulomatous disease in common variable immunodeficiency: a case report and review of the literature. Ann Allergy Asthma Immunol 2005;95(3): 293–300.
109. Quinti I, Agostini C, Tabolli S, et al. Malignancies are the major cause of death in patients with adult onset common variable immunodeficiency. Blood 2012; 120(9):1953–4.
110. Kinlen LJ, Webster AD, Bird AG, et al. Prospective study of cancer in patients with hypogammaglobulinaemia. Lancet 1985;1(8423):263–6.
111. Vajdic CM, Mao L, van Leeuwen MT, et al. Are antibody deficiency disorders associated with a narrower range of cancers than other forms of immunodeficiency? Blood 2010;116(8):1228–34.
112. Bloom KA, Chung D, Cunningham-Rundles C. Osteoarticular infectious complications in patients with primary immunodeficiencies. Curr Opin Rheumatol 2008; 20(4):480–5.
113. Lee AH, Levinson AI, Schumacher HR. Hypogammaglobulinemia and rheumatic disease. Semin Arthritis Rheum 1993;22(4):252–64.
114. Swierkot J, Lewandowicz-Uszynska A, Chlebicki A, et al. Rheumatoid arthritis in a patient with common variable immunodeficiency: difficulty in diagnosis and therapy. Clin Rheumatol 2006;25(1):92–4.
115. Xiao X, Miao Q, Chang C, et al. Common variable immunodeficiency and autoimmunity-an inconvenient truth. Autoimmun Rev 2014;13(8):858–64.
116. Agarwal S, Cunningham-Rundles C. Autoimmunity in common variable immunodeficiency. Curr Allergy Asthma Rep 2009;9(5):347–52.
117. Lucas M, Lee M, Lortan J, et al. Infection outcomes in patients with common variable immunodeficiency disorders: relationship to immunoglobulin therapy over 22 years. J Allergy Clin Immunol 2010;125(6):1354–60.e4.
118. Orange JS, Grossman WJ, Navickis RJ, et al. Impact of trough IgG on pneumonia incidence in primary immunodeficiency: A meta-analysis of clinical studies. Clin Immunol 2010;137(1):21–30.

119. Ballow M. Optimizing immunoglobulin treatment for patients with primary immunodeficiency disease to prevent pneumonia and infection incidence: review of the current data. Ann Allergy Asthma Immunol 2013;111(6 Suppl):S2–5.
120. Castigli E, Wilson S, Garibyan L, et al. Reexamining the role of TACI coding variants in common variable immunodeficiency and selective IgA deficiency. Nat Genet 2007;39(4):430–1.
121. Pan-Hammarström Q, Salzer U, Du L, et al. Reexamining the role of TACI coding variants in common variable immunodeficiency and selective IgA deficiency. Nat Genet 2007;39(4):429–30.
122. Salzer U, Bacchelli C, Buckridge S, et al. Relevance of biallelic versus monoallelic TNFRSF13B mutations in distinguishing disease-causing from risk-increasing TNFRSF13B variants in antibody deficiency syndromes. Blood 2009;113(9):1967–76.
123. Martinez-Pomar N, Detkova D, Aróstegui JI, et al. Role of TNFRSF13B variants in patients with common variable immunodeficiency. Blood 2009;114(13):2846–8.
124. Martinez-Gallo M, Radigan L, Almejún MB, et al. TACI mutations and impaired B-cell function in subjects with CVID and healthy heterozygotes. J Allergy Clin Immunol 2013;131(2):468–76.

Specific Antibody Deficiencies

Luke A. Wall, MD*, Victoria R. Dimitriades, MD, Ricardo U. Sorensen, MD

KEYWORDS

- Specific antibody deficiency • Pneumococcal polysaccharide vaccine
- Recurrent sinopulmonary infections • Vaccine failure • Immunoglobulin replacement

KEY POINTS

- Specific antibody deficiency (SAD) is characterized by failure of response to polysaccharide antigens, with otherwise intact immunity.
- Immunologic challenge with the 23-valent pneumococcal polysaccharide vaccine is currently used as the gold standard for diagnosis.
- SAD encompasses multiple phenotypes, including mild, moderate, severe, and poor immunologic memory.
- Without appropriate diagnosis and treatment, permanent sequelae such as bronchiectasis may occur. Appropriate management allows most patients to achieve a normal life.
- Management options include additional vaccinations, antibiotics, and immunoglobulin replacement.

INTRODUCTION

Specific antibody deficiency (SAD), also known as selective polysaccharide antibody deficiency, is a common primary immunodeficiency disease (PIDD) of the B-cell compartment. Defined as an insufficient antibody response to polysaccharide antigens, evaluation of response to the 23-valent pneumococcal polysaccharide vaccine (PPV23) is the current diagnostic gold standard. Using a pure polysaccharide challenge allows a true assessment of the B-cell compartment, whereas challenge with a protein or protein conjugate vaccine elicits a maximal helper T-cell response. PPV23 has the advantage that a high number of serotypes are included, disallowing a diagnosis based on a single antigen response. It is essential to recognize that

Section of Allergy Immunology, Department of Pediatrics, Louisiana State University Health Sciences Center, Jeffrey Modell Center for Primary Immunodeficiencies, 200 Henry Clay Avenue, New Orleans, LA 70118, USA
* Corresponding author.
E-mail address: lwall@lsuhsc.edu

Immunol Allergy Clin N Am 35 (2015) 659–670
http://dx.doi.org/10.1016/j.iac.2015.07.003   immunology.theclinics.com

patients with SAD typically have completely intact response to protein antigens, including the protein conjugated vaccines.

Failure of polysaccharide response may be observed as a component of a more global PIDD, as well as in the setting of multiple secondary immunodeficient states (**Box 1**). Such disorders are referred to by the more global diagnosis and are not labeled as SAD. This article focuses on SAD in the strictest definition, as the failure of response to polysaccharide antigens in the setting of recurrent infections with normal immunoglobulin isotypes and normal serologic response to protein antigens in patients 2 years old and older.[1–3]

Clinical manifestations of SAD predominantly include recurrent sinopulmonary infections that are more frequent, severe, or prolonged than infections experienced by individuals with intact immunity. SAD may resolve over time, especially when diagnosed in childhood. However, in some patients the deficiency is lifelong. Four phenotypes exist based on the response to PPV23: mild, moderate, severe, and memory.[3]

The management of SAD, including prevention and treatment of recurrent infections, can be classified into the following broad categories: additional immunization, antibiotic prophylaxis and treatment, and immunoglobulin therapy. With appropriate treatment, most patients have an excellent prognosis.

PATHOPHYSIOLOGY

There is no single immunologic mechanism for SAD. Some patients represent delayed physiologic maturation of the immune system, considering that human infants respond in robust fashion to protein antigens, whereas response to polysaccharides may be suboptimal. Hence, the phenotype of young children who are diagnosed with SAD and subsequently experience resolution over time could be explained by a delay in the normal maturation process. The underlying cause for this delay remains unknown.

Abnormally low or deficient specific antibody responses are found in association with many well-defined PIDDs, some of which are presented in **Box 1**.[4] Although these PIDDs with weak polysaccharide response are not classified as SAD per se, they do highlight that a wide spectrum of inborn immunologic defects may lead to a common functional defect manifested by impaired polysaccharide antigen response and susceptibility to sinopulmonary infections.

SAD has been associated with several other subtle immunologic findings. For example, association of SAD with immunoglobulin (Ig) G subclass deficiencies,

---

Box 1
Primary immunodeficiencies and secondary immunodeficient states that may be associated with impaired vaccine response

Primary	Acquired
Wiskott-Aldrich syndrome	Splenectomy
DiGeorge syndrome	Immunosuppression
Asplenia	Malnutrition
Hyper–immunoglobulin E (Job) syndrome	Protein-losing enteropathy
Common variable immune deficiency	Nephrotic syndrome
Dock8 deficiency	Chylothorax
NEMO deficiency	Human immunodeficiency virus infection
Class switch recombination defects	—
Selective immunoglobulin A deficiency	—
Immunoglobulin G subclass deficiency	—

particularly IgG2 deficiency, has been described.[5] Typically, IgG2 subclass–deficient patients develop protective antibody titers to a restricted number of serotypes in the pneumococcal polysaccharide vaccine. These patients often have poor immunologic memory, with titers decreasing to preimmunization levels several months following vaccination.[6] Although such associations may offer important clues to the pathophysiologic mechanisms of SAD, details remain elusive despite years of research.

Regarding susceptibility to infection among patients with SAD, pathogens are not restricted to *Streptococcus pneumoniae*. Other encapsulated bacterial pathogens, such as *Haemophilus influenzae* and *Moraxella catarrhalis*, are common. *Staphylococcus aureus* and respiratory viruses also cause significant infections in patients with SAD.[7] This observation emphasizes that the presence of SAD represents a more general dysfunction of antibody-mediated immunity, rather than susceptibility to a specific pathogen.

EPIDEMIOLOGY

Although prevalence in the general population is not well established, up to 15% of children undergoing evaluation for recurrent infections are diagnosed with SAD.[8] Among all PIDDs treated in the immunology clinic, SAD accounted for at least 23% of all diagnoses in a review of a referral center in the United States.[9] A recent study from the United Kingdom reported diagnosis of SAD in 58% of children who underwent evaluation for chronic wet cough with duration of greater than 8 weeks.[10]

SAD may also be diagnosed in adolescents and adults. In a recent study, 12% of adults with refractory chronic rhinosinusitis met diagnostic criteria for SAD.[11]

NATURAL HISTORY

Among children with SAD, symptoms and immunologic findings may improve with age. Roughly half of children show resolution of SAD within 3 years. Treatment is often required, but may be temporary (1–2 years).[12] Permanent sequelae or organ damage secondary to infections is rare among such children if treatment is instituted appropriately.

A new diagnosis of SAD outside of childhood could either represent a previously missed diagnosis or progression of a previously mild immunologic phenotype. Adolescent and adult patients require close attention, because they may have already developed bronchiectasis and SAD is less likely to resolve over time in this age group. A subset of adults and adolescents with SAD may experience progression to more severe forms of PIDD, including hypogammaglobulinemia and common variable immunodeficiency.[7]

SYMPTOMS

The signs and symptoms of SAD are similar to those of other antibody deficiency syndromes. Common manifestations include chronic and recurrent otitis media, sinusitis, bronchitis, and pneumonia. Infections are more frequent, severe, or prolonged than those experienced by normal individuals. A common pattern is partial or temporary improvement with antibiotic therapy, followed by a rapid return of infections on discontinuation of antibiotics. In the United States, less than 5% of patients with SAD experience invasive infections.[12] This relative absence of life-threatening infections is not surprising because antibiotics are prescribed commonly in the general population, early in the course of infection. Nonetheless, patients who have not been appropriately identified and treated may present with bronchiectasis or severe refractory sinusitis.[11,13]

For a common childhood infection such as otitis media, characteristics frequently found in patients with SAD include:

- Early onset of infections, as early as 3 to 4 months of age
- Recurrence of infection after antibiotic treatment
- Recurrence after tympanostomy tube placement
- Need for replacement of tympanostomy tubes multiple times

It is common for patients with SAD to also present with symptoms resembling atopic diseases, including rhinitis and asthma. One study reported asthma in 58% and rhinitis in 55% of children with SAD.[12] Only some of these patients have a well-documented IgE-mediated allergic sensitization. It is important to consider that patients with allergic symptoms experience inflammation of the nasopharynx leading to impaired sinus cavity drainage and eustachian tube dysfunction, which can lead to sinopulmonary infections. Patients with SAD who fit this clinical description are among the most challenging to identify because sinopulmonary infections may be blamed solely on allergic symptoms of rhinitis and asthma. Astute clinicians may use several clues, listed in **Box 2**, to determine when an evaluation for antibody deficiency is appropriate among such patients.

DIAGNOSTIC EVALUATION
Initial Approach to the Patient

The initial evaluation of a patient with an abnormal pattern of sinopulmonary infections must include a detailed history and physical examination focused on the pattern of infections, documentation of any pathogens previously isolated, and consideration of any permanent sequelae. At a minimum, a complete blood cell count with differential, immunoglobulin isotypes (IgG, IgA, IgM, and IgE), and baseline pneumococcal serotype–specific IgG antibody titers should be obtained. Immunization with PPV23 during the first clinic visit is optional in patients who have a highly convincing clinical history, as long as baseline titers are ordered the same day. A local vaccine reaction (Arthus reaction) is possible in patients who already have high antipneumococcal antibodies. For this reason, many clinicians opt to administer PPV23 at the second clinic visit, after the baseline pneumococcal titer results are available. Following PPV23 administration, titers should be repeated by the same laboratory in 4 to 8 weeks.

PPV23 is typically not administered to patients who have high titers to most serotypes at baseline. This approach applies to patients who have high titers despite being

---

Box 2
Helpful hints: when to suspect an antibody defect among patients with presumed allergic rhinosinusitis and/or asthma

Frequent purulent nasal discharge

Failure to identify allergic triggers (negative allergy testing)

Little improvement with allergy treatment and allergen avoidance

Chest symptoms do not improve with inhaled bronchodilators

Frequent wet cough (as opposed to classic dry cough of asthma)

Absence of itchy, watery eyes

Infrequent sneezing and itching of the nose

Transient improvement with antibiotic treatment

pneumococcal conjugate vaccine (PCV) naive, as well as those who have received PCV and have protective titers to PCV and non-PCV serotypes. Such patients who have developed high titers in response to natural infection, but maintain an abnormal pattern of infections, should be considered for other forms of PIDD as well as other causes for recurrent infections such as mucociliary or anatomic defects.

Laboratory Considerations Regarding Antipneumococcal Antibody Titers

Although a variety of panels are available commercially with varying numbers of serotypes, most immunologists include at least 14 serotype-specific IgG antipneumococcal antibody titers. It is optimal for the panel to include at least 7 PPV23-exclusive serotypes, present only in the PPV23 and absent in the conjugated vaccine that was previously administered (**Table 1**). Completion of the 13-valent conjugate vaccine (PCV13) series is recommended in young children before challenge with PPV23. Therefore, measurement of PPV23-exclusive serotypes is necessary in evaluating the PPV23 response.[14,15]

Table 1
Serotypes contained in pneumococcal vaccines

Serotypes	Vaccines		
	PPV23	PCV7	PCV13
1	X	—	X
2	X	—	—
3	X	—	X
4	X	X	X
5	X	—	X
6A	—	—	X
6B	X	X	X
7F	X	—	X
8	X	—	—
9N	X	—	—
9V	X	X	X
10A	X	—	—
11A	X	—	—
12F	X	—	—
14	X	X	X
15B	X	—	—
17F	X	—	—
18C	X	X	X
19A	X	—	X
19F	X	X	X
20	X	—	—
22F	X	—	—
23F	X	X	X
33F	X	—	—

Abbreviations: PCV7, heptavalent conjugate vaccine; PCV13, 13-valent conjugate vaccine.
  Courtesy of R.U. Sorensen, MD, New Orleans, LA.

For IgG serotype–specific antipneumococcal antibody assessment, the standard method is the third-generation World Health Organization enzyme-linked immunosorbent assay (ELISA), which incorporates double absorption of samples with capsular polysaccharide and serotype 22F. This technique increases specificity by removing nonspecific antibodies.[16–18] Commercial laboratories have now adopted measurement of specific antibodies using Luminex. Results with this test vary from those obtained by ELISA. Clinical validation of the usefulness of Luminex is still in progress.[18,19]

PPV23 has the advantage that a high number of serotypes are included, disallowing a diagnosis based on a single antigen response. Measurement of total antipneumococcal IgG in a single test that produces 1 numeric value without differentiating specific antibodies to individual serotypes is not useful. It is common for patients with SAD to develop an increased titer to a limited number of serotypes, whereas most serotypes remain nonprotective. Such a pattern cannot be elucidated by a test that does not distinguish between serotypes.

Although serotype-specific titers as low as 0.35 µg/mL have been considered to be protective against invasive infections, a titer of 1.3 µg/mL is generally considered protective against mucosal infections and is used as the threshold of response to PPV23.[3,20,21]

Interpretation of the Pneumococcal Polysaccharide Response

By 2 years of age, most individuals have developed protective titers to at least some serotypes in response to natural infection. Hence, the absence of protective antibodies to all serotypes tested at baseline is unusual, even in nonimmunized patients. By current definitions, low antibody concentrations following natural infection, or following PCV administration, do not specifically define a SAD phenotype unless there is a subsequent inadequate response to PPV23.

When gauging a sufficient PPV23 response for an individual patient, one approach in the past has been to compare postimmunization serotype-specific antibody concentrations with preimmunization concentrations, considering normal to be a 4-fold increase in the concentration. Other sources accept a 2-fold increase. This approach is no longer favored, because it involves at least 2 major pitfalls. First, if the baseline titer is greater than 4 µg/mL, individuals with intact immunity may not produce a significant increase in titer on vaccine challenge[22]; the higher the baseline titer to an individual serotype, the less likely a significant increase is in the setting of a normal immune response.[2,3] The second downfall to this approach is that, if a baseline titer to an individual serotype is exceedingly low, even with an increase of several fold, the post-PPV23 titer may remain less than the protective range. Such low post-PPV23 titers indicate a failed response.

Most experts now agree that the most reliable and straightforward approach in gauging response to PPV23 is to consider the percentage of serotype-specific titers measured (titers to serotypes included in PPV23) that are within the protective range post-PPV23. Note that with this approach to interpretation the final enumeration of serotypes to which protective titers have developed may include a combination of titers that are achieved through natural infection, as well as those achieved following PPV23 administration. An acceptable percentage of protective serotypes is greater than or equal to 50% of serotypes for patients less than 6 years of age, and greater than or equal to 70% of serotypes of patients aged greater than or equal to 6 years. This approach assumes that an individual serotype is considered protective at a value of greater than or equal to 1.3 µg/mL. This straightforward recommendation adds a much-needed simplicity to the evaluation process. When assessing patients who have previously received PCV, the most consistent and straightforward approach is to focus solely on the PPV23-exclusive serotypes, which were not included in the PCV that was previously administered.[23] Considering all of the aforementioned factors, the approach to the interpretation of response to PPV23 is summarized as follows:

- Patients who are PCV naive:
  - Among all PPV23 serotype titers measured, the percentage of these serotypes that are in the protective range post-PPV23 is considered the percentage response.
- Patients who have previously received PCV:
  - At least 7 PPV23-exclusive serotypes should be measured.
  - The evaluation may be based solely on the PPV23-exclusive serotypes.
  - Among all PPV23-exclusive serotypes measured, the percentage of these that are in the protective range post-PPV23 is considered the percentage response.

Diagnosis of Specific Antibody Deficiency Phenotypes

Four defined phenotypes of SAD are currently accepted based on the antibody response to individual PPV23 serotypes: mild, moderate, severe, and memory (**Table 2**). All phenotypes assume an abnormal pattern of infection.[3] It is essential to recognize that these phenotypes refer exclusively to characteristics of the serologic diagnosis, and may or may not correlate with the clinical severity or degree of susceptibility to infections for an individual patient.

- Severe phenotype, defined as nearly absent response to pneumococcal polysaccharides, is the most straightforward to diagnose. These patients have protective titers to less than or equal to 2 serotypes following PPV23.[3,6] The clinical susceptibility to infections is typically severe as well.
- Moderate phenotype is defined based on age at the time of PPV23 administration:
  - Age less than 6 years: less than 50% of serotypes protective
  - Age greater than or equal to 6 years: less than 70% of serotypes protective
- Mild phenotype is less well defined. However, many patients with significant infections are in this category. Considering that most normal individuals have a robust response to most PPV23 serotypes, mild SAD can be defined in the broadest sense as failure of response to multiple serotypes.

Table 2
Summary of SAD phenotypes based on PPV23 response

Phenotype	Age ≥6 y	Age <6 y	Notes
Severe	≤2 protective titers	≤2 protective titers	Protective titers present are low
Moderate	<70% of serotypes protective	<50% of serotypes protective	Protective titers present to ≥3 serotypes
Mild	Failure to generate protective titers to multiple serotypes	Failure to generate protective titers to multiple serotypes	—
Memory	Loss of response within 6 mo	Loss of response within 6 mo	Adequate initial response

Note that all phenotypes assume a history of infections.
Protective level refers to greater than or equal to 1.3 µg/mL.
Adapted from Orange J, Ballow M, Stiehm ER, et al. Use and interpretation of diagnostic vaccination in primary immunodeficiency: a working group report of the Basic and Clinical Immunology Interest Section of the American Academy of Allergy, Asthma & Immunology. J Allergy Clin Immunol 2012;130(3 Suppl):S14; with permission.

- Memory phenotype is defined by an adequate initial response (based on age) with subsequent loss of titers within 6 months.

MANAGEMENT

Management must always be tailored based on the clinical severity of infections. Overall, the management of patients who have failed to respond serologically to PPV23 can be grouped into the following broad categories: additional immunization, antibiotic prophylaxis and treatment, and immunoglobulin therapy.

Immunization

In patients with poor immunologic memory, once antipneumococcal titers wane, reimmunization with PPV23 may result in reestablishing protective antibody levels and increased clinical protection. There is a counterargument against repeated administration of polysaccharide vaccines based on limited, controversial reports that repeated immunization may produce hyporesponsiveness.[24] Most clinicians recommend waiting at least 1 year before administration of a second dose of PPV23, and only consider administration in patients who showed a transient initial response. Multiple, repeat PPV23 administration is not likely to be effective and is not recommended. For patients who showed complete absence of response to an initial dose, there is no indication to administer the vaccine again.

Patients who fail to respond to the initial challenge with PPV23 may respond to the conjugated vaccine. Between 80% and 90% of patients with SAD have a strong serologic response to PCV.[2] Therefore, the pneumococcal conjugate vaccine containing the largest number of serotypes currently available (PCV13) should be considered in patients who have failed PPV23 and may produce clinical benefit. However, even if the serologic PCV response is robust, such patients must be approached with caution because they have previously shown polysaccharide response failure and may not respond normally to natural infections with encapsulated organisms.

There is also evidence that PCV may prime the response to a subsequent dose of PPV23. Therefore, if patients have failed to respond to PPV23 at the initial evaluation and subsequently receive a PCV dose based on the aforementioned approach, but maintain an abnormal pattern of infection, reimmunization with PPV23 after 1 year may produce a better response by taking advantage of the priming effect of the conjugate vaccine.[14,25] This approach may be more practical in patients who were truly naive to pneumococcal vaccines at the time of their initial evaluation.

Antibiotics

Antibiotic prophylaxis should be considered, especially in young patients who are likely to outgrow SAD. When an oral antibiotic is considered for prophylaxis, trimethoprim-sulfamethoxazole or amoxicillin can be effective. Use of intranasal mupirocin ointment, applied daily for several months to a year, is a safe adjunct prophylactic measure.

Appropriate antibiotic treatment of any bacterial respiratory infection is important. Treatment with high doses of antibiotics for a period of at least 2 weeks is necessary. When antibiotic use alone improves the patient's quality of life and prevents infectious complications, no additional treatment is needed. Note that patients with SAD who are excessively and/or chronically infected may have been previously treated with many antibiotics. Such patients may warrant imaging for complicated chronic sinusitis or bronchiectasis, based on the clinical manifestations, and treatment of any identified chronic infection. For such patients, prophylaxis may be futile because of infection and colonization with multiple antibiotic-resistant organisms. Implementation of immunoglobulin replacement, without a trial of antibiotic prophylaxis, may be appropriate in such clinically severe patients.

Immunoglobulin Replacement Therapy

Immunoglobulin replacement is indicated for patients with mild, moderate, or memory phenotypes who experience persistent infections despite appropriate management. Furthermore, patients with the severe phenotype may be placed directly on immunoglobulin replacement. Immunoglobulin replacement may prevent complications such as hearing loss, sinus damage, and bronchiectasis while significantly affecting quality of life and reducing the need for excessive medical visits and missed work/school. Patients with any form of SAD who have already developed permanent organ damage, such as bronchiectasis, should be placed directly on immunoglobulin replacement, because other treatment options are likely to fail.

The recommended immunoglobulin starting dose is at least 400 to 600 mg/kg/month. Immunoglobulin can be given intravenously once monthly. In addition, several subcutaneous immunoglobulin options are available with various techniques and intervals. Patients who experience repeated breakthrough infections or have bronchiectasis require higher doses and/or shorter intervals between doses.

When immunoglobulin replacement is initiated, patients should be advised that treatment will be discontinued after a period of 1 to 2 years and the immune response will be reevaluated 4 to 6 months after discontinuation of immunoglobulin replacement. The discontinuation of immunoglobulin should be scheduled during the spring or summer seasons, when the incidence of infections typically decreases. As an exception to this approach, adults and adolescents with the severe phenotype and patients with permanent organ damage should continue to receive immunoglobulin infusion indefinitely, without the need for such reevaluation.

Six months after the final immunoglobulin dose, a complete evaluation of antibody-mediated immunity should be repeated. If the pneumococcal titers are again low, an additional dose of PPV23 should be administered followed by measurement of post-PPV23 titers 4 weeks after immunization. Many children do not require further immunoglobulin replacement therapy, but some continue to have persistent infections and need to resume the infusions. These patients are likely to have additional immunologic abnormalities that are presently under evaluation.

Some patients experience a significant recurrence of infections soon after discontinuation of immunoglobulin therapy. Such patients have proved, based on clinical grounds alone, that their diagnosis of SAD has not resolved. Immunoglobulin therapy should be reinstituted for such patients based on a significant recurrence of infections, without waiting 6 months for the repeat laboratory evaluation. Patient management, immunoglobulin replacement therapy, and posttreatment evaluation can be complex and are best served by experts in the management of patients with PIDD.

PROGNOSIS

The immunologic phenotypes of SAD may be transient or permanent. Transient forms are more common in children 2 to 5 years of age. Even in permanent phenotypes, the prognosis of patients with SAD is good with proper management. Undiagnosed or improperly treated patients may develop permanent sequelae.

Patients who outgrow SAD should continue to be monitored, because it has not been determined whether such patients will face immunologic problems later in life. These patients should be seen in clinic at least annually and educated to contact the immunologist if an abnormal pattern of infection returns.

In particular, older patients with selective antibody deficiencies should be monitored closely, because they may eventually develop common variable immunodeficiency.

FUTURE CONSIDERATIONS

The current era of research regarding the specific antibody deficiencies is promising. Immunologic markers, including IgM memory and class-switched memory B cells, are providing additional depth to the understanding of SAD.[26] It is expected that such markers in combination with large-scale DNA studies, correlated with detailed clinical patterns, will soon produce clinically relevant information that will aid in determining the diagnosis, treatment, and prognosis for individual patients with SAD.

There is a need for clinical correlation of laboratory tests that can determine the functional capacity of antibodies. Opsonophagocytic assays are cumbersome and have not been widely validated clinically. Avidity testing to individual pneumococcal serotypes is now available commercially. This test could be helpful in unique situations, such as when a patient manifests a severe pattern of sinopulmonary infections but challenge with PPV23 produces high antipneumococcal antibody titers. Such titers could be of robust levels, but they might not be functioning optimally. Much remains to be learned regarding such tests and their clinical application.

Additional phenotypes, which are already observed clinically, will undoubtedly come into acceptance as they are described in immunologic and clinical detail. For example, we have observed several children who manifest abnormal immunologic memory but do not strictly fit within the current diagnostic criteria. These patients show a robust response to PPV23, maintain titers at 6 months, but go on to experience complete loss of titers for essentially all serotypes with recurrence of infections by 12 to 18 months following PPV23. A cohort of such patients with the most impressive pattern of infections has been treated at our center with immunoglobulin replacement, which has produced drastic improvement. This group of patients is not currently well described in the literature. Perhaps these patients represent a second immunologic memory phenotype, in which memory wanes much faster than in the average population, but not as rapidly as 6 months.

Another group that deserves closer attention is the cohort of patients who completely fail to mount a serologic response to the 4-dose PCV series in childhood, which is not currently considered pathologic. Some clinicians argue that failure to develop antipneumococcal antibodies to all serotypes contained in PCV should be considered pathologic in a child with recurrent infections, regardless of subsequent response to PPV23. This entity has been proposed as PCV-SAD. More studies are needed in this group of patients with impaired antibody response.[26]

Little is known about the long-term outcome of patients who are diagnosed with SAD at a young age and subsequently improve over time. Long-term studies are needed in this group of patients to determine the risk for immunologic derangements later in life.

SUMMARY

SAD is a group of antibody defects characterized by failure of immunologic response to polysaccharide antigens in the setting of recurrent sinopulmonary infections with otherwise intact immunity. SAD represents a group of disorders with a wide spectrum of clinical and immunologic phenotypes. Although permanent organ damage such as bronchiectasis is possible, most patients do well with appropriate treatment. Caution is strongly advised regarding the approach to patients who may fit a mild phenotype, or have a borderline diagnosis, but manifest a significant pattern of infections.

Because immunologic severity does not correlate with clinical severity in many patients, treatment should be tailored based on the clinical manifestations of the patient.

REFERENCES

1. Sanders LA, Rijkers GT, Kuis W, et al. Defective antipneumococcal polysaccharide antibody response in children with recurrent respiratory tract infections. J Allergy Clin Immunol 1993;91(1 Pt 1):110–9.
2. Sorensen RU, Leiva LE, Javier FC 3rd, et al. Influence of age on the response to *Streptococcus pneumoniae* vaccine in patients with recurrent infections and normal immunoglobulin concentrations. J Allergy Clin Immunol 1998;102(2):215–21.
3. Orange J, Ballow M, Stiehm ER, et al. Use and interpretation of diagnostic vaccination in primary immunodeficiency: a working group report of the Basic and Clinical Immunology Interest Section of the American Academy of Allergy, Asthma & Immunology. J Allergy Clin Immunol 2012;130(3 Suppl):S1–24.
4. Knutsen A. Patients with IgG subclass and/or selective antibody deficiency to polysaccharide antigens: initiation of a controlled clinical trial of intravenous immune globulin. J Allergy Clin Immunol 1989;84:640.
5. Bernatowska-Matuszkiewicz E, Pac M, Pum M, et al. IgG subclasses and antibody response to pneumococcal capsular polysaccharides in children with severe sinopulmonary infections and asthma. Immunol Invest 1991;20:173.
6. Sorensen R, Hidalgo H, Moore C, et al. Anti-pneumococcal antibody titers and IgG subclasses in children with recurrent respiratory infections. Pediatr Pulmonol 1996;22:167.
7. Knutsen A. Spectrum of antibody deficiency disorders with normal or near-normal immunoglobulin levels. Pediatr Asthma Allergy Immunol 2006;19(1):51–62.
8. Boyle RJ, Le C, Balloch A, et al. The clinical syndrome of specific antibody deficiency in children. Clin Exp Immunol 2006;146(3):486–92.
9. Javier F, Moore C, Sorensen R. Distribution of primary immunodeficiency diseases diagnosed in a pediatric tertiary hospital. Ann Allergy Asthma Immunol 2000;84:25.
10. Lim MT, Jeyarajah K, Jones P, et al. Specific antibody deficiency in children with chronic wet cough. Arch Dis Child 2012;97(5):478–80.
11. Carr TF, Koterba AP, Chandra R, et al. Characterization of specific antibody deficiency in adults with medically refractory chronic rhinosinusitis. Am J Rhinol Allergy 2011;25(4):241–4.
12. Wolpert J, Knutsen A. Natural history of selective antibody deficiency to bacterial polysaccharide antigens in children. Pediatr Asthma Allergy Immunol 1998;12:183–91.
13. Vendrell M, de Gracia J, Rodrigo MJ, et al. Antibody production deficiency with normal IgG levels in bronchiectasis of unknown etiology. Chest 2005;127(1):197–204.
14. Rose MA, Schubert R, Strnad N, et al. Priming of immunological memory by pneumococcal conjugate vaccine in children unresponsive to 23-valent polysaccharide pneumococcal vaccine. Clin Diagn Lab Immunol 2005;12(10):1216–22.
15. Paris K, Sorensen R. Assessment and clinical interpretation of polysaccharide antibody responses. Ann Allergy Asthma Immunol 2007;99:462–4.
16. Concepcion N, Frasch C. Pneumococcal type 22f polysaccharide absorption improves the specificity of a pneumococcal-polysaccharide enzyme-linked immunosorbent assay. Clin Diagn Lab Immunol 2001;8:266–72.

17. Henckaerts I, Goldblatt D, Ashton L, et al. Critical differences between pneumococcal polysaccharide enzyme-linked immunosorbent assays with and without 22F inhibition at low antibody concentrations in pediatric sera. Clin Vaccine Immunol 2006;13(3):356–60.
18. Balloch A, Licciardi PV, Tang ML. Serotype-specific anti-pneumococcal IgG and immune competence: critical differences in interpretation criteria when different methods are used. J Clin Immunol 2013;33(2):335–41.
19. Sorensen RU, Leiva LE. Measurement of pneumococcal polysaccharide antibodies. J Clin Immunol 2014;34(2):127–8.
20. Black S, Eskola J, Whitney C, et al. Pneumococcal conjugate vaccine and pneumococcal common protein vaccines. In: Plotkin SA, Orenstein WA, Offit PA, editors. Vaccines. Philadelphia: Saunders Elsevier; 2008. p. 531–67.
21. Siber G, Chang I, Baker S, et al. Estimating the protective concentration of anti-pneumococcal capsular polysaccharide antibodies. Vaccine 2007;25(19):3816–26.
22. Hare ND, Smith BJ, Ballas ZK. Antibody response to pneumococcal vaccination as a function of preimmunization titer. J Allergy Clin Immunol 2009;123(1):195–200.
23. Leiva L, Sorensen RU. Selective antibody deficiency with normal immunoglobulins. In: Sullivan KE, Stiehm ER, editors. Stiehm's immune deficiencies. San Diego: Elsevier; 2014. p. 409–16.
24. Granoff DM, Gupta RK, Belshe RB, et al. Induction of immunologic refractoriness in adults by meningococcal C polysaccharide vaccination. J Infect Dis 1998;178(3):870–4.
25. Sorensen RU, Leiva LE, Giangrosso PA, et al. Response to a heptavalent conjugate Streptococcus pneumoniae vaccine in children with recurrent infections who are unresponsive to the polysaccharide vaccine. Pediatr Infect Dis J 1998;17(8):685–91.
26. Leiva L, Monjure H, Sorensen R. Recurrent respiratory infections, specific antibody deficiencies, and memory B cells. J Clin Immunol 2013;33:S57–61.

Severe Combined Immunodeficiency Disorders

Ivan K. Chinn, MD*, William T. Shearer, MD, PhD

KEYWORDS

- Severe combined immunodeficiency disease • DiGeorge anomaly • Transplantation
- Gene therapy • Newborn screening

KEY POINTS

- Severe combined immunodeficiency disease (SCID) is defined by (1) the absence or very low number of T cells (<300 CD3 T cells/mm^3) and no or very low T-cell function (<10% of the lower limit of normal) as measured by response to phytohemagglutinin (PHA) or (2) the presence of T cells of maternal origin.
- Fourteen molecular defects are recognized as causing SCID: *IL2RG, JAK3, RAG1, RAG2, DCLRE1C, PRKDC, IL7R, CD3D, CD3E, CD247, PTPRC, CORO1A, ADA,* and *AK2.* Several others are often considered to be associated with SCID as well.
- Definitive treatment options for SCID include hematopoietic bone marrow stem cell transplant or gene therapy. Transplant before 3.5 months of age remains essential for optimal survival and immune reconstitution. Conditioning should not be used in patients with active infections.
- Complete DiGeorge anomaly produces a T-negative, B-positive, natural killer (NK)-positive phenotype that can be confused with SCID. It is diagnosed clinically and cannot be excluded by negative genetic testing results. Allogeneic thymus transplantation provides the optimal long-term solution for complete DiGeorge anomaly but remains limited in availability.
- Newborn screening for SCID has proved highly successful in identifying infants with SCID and complete DiGeorge anomaly. It has demonstrated that the incidence of SCID in the United States is 1 per 58,000 live births and has led to life-saving treatment of affected children.

INTRODUCTION

Severe combined immunodeficiency disorders are characterized by a lack of protective T-, B-, and sometimes NK-cell responses to infections. As a result, affected individuals are born with marked susceptibility to pathogens that ultimately cannot be

Disclosures: Drs I.K. Chinn and W.T. Shearer have no conflicts of interest to disclose.
Section of Immunology, Allergy, and Rheumatology, Department of Pediatrics, Texas Children's Hospital, Baylor College of Medicine, 1102 Bates Avenue, Suite 330, Houston, TX 77030-2399, USA
* Corresponding author.
E-mail address: chinn@bcm.edu

Immunol Allergy Clin N Am 35 (2015) 671–694
http://dx.doi.org/10.1016/j.iac.2015.07.002
0889-8561/15/$ – see front matter © 2015 Elsevier Inc. All rights reserved.

managed or controlled. Infection-related death typically occurs by 1 to 2 years of age in the absence of treatment. Thus, these disorders represent true pediatric emergencies.

Failure to generate T cells can result from either intrinsic defects in T-cell precursors that preclude their survival or from absence of the thymic environment necessary for thymocytes to properly mature into naive T cells. The former condition is broadly categorized into a condition known as SCID. The latter condition, congenital athymia, occurs in children with complete DiGeorge anomaly or, more rarely, *FOXN1* deficiency.

This article reviews both SCID and congenital athymia. For SCID, acknowledgment is given to the fact that increased screening of newborns for the condition in the United States quickly brings affected infants to the attention of medical providers, who must then counsel family members regarding options for treatment and anticipated prognosis. Thus, although some of the more common known molecular causes of SCID in North America are discussed, emphasis is placed on conditions that merit special therapeutic considerations, key clinical evaluations, and various approaches toward definitive therapy. For congenital athymia, complete DiGeorge anomaly and *FOXN1* deficiency are reviewed, including typical and atypical presentations. Treatment modalities are then presented. Finally, newborn screening for severe combined immunodeficiency disorders is discussed, including its utility and particular challenges that physicians may face when presented with abnormal results.

Severe Combined Immunodeficiency Disease

Definition

Because combined immunodeficiency diseases, which often do not require immediate correction, are sometimes mistaken for or misdiagnosed as SCID, criteria have been adopted by the Primary Immune Deficiency Treatment Consortium (PIDTC) to define the severe phenotype. Initial guidelines stated that in the absence of an established genetic defect, minimum criteria should include negative human immunodeficiency virus testing and at least 2 of the following 3 conditions: (1) Marked lymphocytopenia and/or T-cell (CD3) lymphopenia (based on age-appropriate reference ranges), (2) severe defect in T-cell proliferation to mitogens (<10% of the lower limit of the reference/normal response), and (3) marked decrease in thymic function (decreased/absent CD4$^+$CD45RA$^+$ naive T cells or T-cell receptor rearrangement excision circles).[1] Subsequently, the criteria were revised to define typical SCID as (1) absence or very low number of T cells (<300 CD3 T cells/mm^3) and no or very low T-cell function (<10% of the lower limit of normal) as measured by response to PHA or (2) presence of T cells of maternal origin.[2] Thus, enumeration of naive T cells or recent thymic emigrants remains important but not essential. These current criteria should be used to establish a diagnosis for clinical and research purposes.

Molecular defects

The first molecular cause of a primary immunodeficiency disease was identified in 1972 when Dr Robert A. Good serendipitously discovered that lack of adenosine deaminase (ADA) results in SCID. Clinical immunologists continued to puzzle, however, over the fact that ADA deficiency is inherited in an autosomal recessive pattern, but children with SCID are nonetheless predominantly boys. The next molecular cause of SCID would not be identified for another 3 decades, when investigators demonstrated that defects in *IL2RG* cause X-linked SCID.[3,4] With the development of advanced molecular cloning techniques and complete sequencing of the human genome, discoveries of the genetic causes of SCID rapidly progressed. Now, at least 14 molecular defects have been confirmed to cause SCID.[5]

Although technological advances[6] will eventually make rapid identification of genetic defects in patients with SCID less challenging for medical providers (**Table 1**), understanding of some of the common causes of SCID remains warranted because of potential implications for management, prognosis, or genetic counseling of family members. Traditionally, characterization of the absence or presence of B and NK cells has permitted clinicians to focus attention toward certain genetic defects (**Table 2**). This system continues to provide value in terms of laying a foundation for understanding several of the fundamental pathogenic mechanisms that cause SCID.

B-positive, natural killer–negative severe combined immunodeficiency disease

This immunologic phenotype is generally caused by molecular defects that are capable of negatively affecting development of both T and NK cells. One likely explanation, then, might involve a defect in a protein shared by T- and NK-cell cytokine signaling pathways. As such, the most common cause of B-positive, NK-negative SCID is a defect in *IL2RG*, which encodes the gamma component (γc) of cytokine receptors for interleukin (IL)-2, IL-4, IL-7, IL-9, IL-15, and IL-21.[7,8] The defect in IL-7 signaling results in failure to generate T cells[9]; NK-cell deficiency occurs chiefly because of the defect in IL-15 signaling.[10,11] Patients are able to create B cells because, unlike in mice, IL-7 receptor signaling is dispensable for B-cell development in humans.[9] However, the B cells are unable to produce protective antibody responses because of defective IL-4 receptor signaling.[12] *IL2RG* is located at Xq13. *IL2RG* genetic defects are therefore inherited in an X-linked recessive pattern and account for the male predominance of SCID cases seen in the United States.[13] Although many cases appear spontaneously, testing of the mother for carrier status remains important for genetic counseling purposes. On the other hand, autosomal recessive cases of B-positive, NK-negative SCID are also known to occur, affecting boys and girls equally. Because *IL2RG* is not altered in these children, it would seem reasonable to suspect a defect in a signaling cascade protein downstream from γc. In fact, γc activation leads to phosphorylation of Janus kinase 3 (JAK3), which then mediates further signaling through signal transducer and activator of transcription proteins. Defects in *JAK3* are now known to cause most cases of autosomal recessive B-positive, NK-negative SCID.[14,15]

B-negative, natural killer–positive severe combined immunodeficiency disease

This phenotype immediately raises suspicion for a defect in a process common to both T and B cells but not to NK cells. Accordingly, T and B cells rearrange the DNA that encodes their antigen receptors during their development. This mechanism, known as V(D)J recombination, allows for receptor diversity and specificity toward antigens, yielding adaptive immunity. Unsuccessful V(D)J recombination results in apoptosis. NK cells do not participate in this process, rendering them immune to V(D)J

Table 1

Representative list of genes developed and available at Baylor Medical Center/Texas Children's Hospital for rapid, targeted, high-throughput sequencing to identify newborns who require urgent consultation for transplantation

ADA	AK2	AP3B1	CASP8	CD3D	CD3E	CD3G	CHD7	CD8A	CIITA
CORO1A	DCLRE1C	DOCK8	FOXN1	FOXP3	IKZF1	IL2RG	IL7R	ITK	JAK3
LCK	LIG4	LYST	NHEJ1	ORAI1	PNP	PRF1	PRKDC	PTPRC	RAG1
RAG2	RFX5	RFXANK	RFXAP	RMRP	SH2D1A	STAT5B	STIM1	STX11	STXBP2
TAP1	TBX1	TTC7A	UNC13D	XIAP	ZAP70	—	—	—	—

Table 2
Molecular causes of SCID and SCID-like disorders, as defined by the IUIS expert committee for primary immunodeficiency

Condition	Defect
SCID	
B-positive, NK-negative	*IL2RG*
	JAK3
B-negative, NK-positive	*RAG1*
	RAG2
	DCLRE1C
	PRKDC
B-positive, NK-positive	*IL7R*
	CD3D
	CD3E
	CD247
	PTPRC
	CORO1A
B-negative, NK-negative	*ADA*
	AK2
Non-SCID	
PNP	*PNP*
CD3γ deficiency	*CD3G*
Zeta chain associated protein kinase 70 deficiency	*ZAP70*[146]
MHC class I deficiency	*TAP*[147,148]
MHC class II deficiency[149]	*CIITA*[150]
	RFX-B[151]
	RFXANK[152,153]
	RFX5[154]
	RFXAP[155]
Dedicator of cytokinesis 8 deficiency[156,157]	*DOCK8*[155,156]
P56lck	*LCK*[158,159]
Calcium release activated channel related defects[160]	*ORAI1*[161]
	STIM1[162]
Folate transport defects	*MTHFD1*[163]
	PCFT[164]

Abbreviations: MHC, major histocompatibility complex; PNP, purine nucleoside phosphorylase.

recombination defects. Not surprisingly, most known molecular causes of B-negative, NK-positive SCID involve defects in proteins necessary for V(D)J recombination. Recombination begins when recombinase activating genes 1 (RAG1) and 2 (RAG2), respectively, recognize recombination signal sequences adjacent to V, D, and J segments and cleave the genomic DNA at those sites. The excised DNA forms a circular episome (in T cells known as a T-cell receptor excision circle [TREC]). For the remaining genomic DNA, intrinsic nonhomologous end-joining DNA repair mechanisms are used to complete V(D)J recombination. The free ends of DNA created by RAG1 and RAG2 cleavage are protected by formation of hairpin loops. These loops must be opened by DNA repair proteins Ku 70, Ku 80, PK_{CS}, and Artemis to allow for the ends of the DNA to be reattached to each other. After the loops are opened, DNA ligation occurs with additional recruitment of DNA ligase IV, XRCC4, and XLF (also known as Cernunnos). Most commonly for B-negative, NK-positive SCID, defects are found in *RAG1* or *RAG2*, followed by *DCLRE1C*, which encodes Artemis.[16,17] Mutations in PK_{CS},[18,19]

DNA ligase IV,[20–22] and Cernunnos[23] have also been reported to cause SCID but do not commonly occur in the United States. SCID-causing defects in Ku 70, Ku 80, and XRCC4 have not yet been observed in humans.

B-positive, natural killer–positive severe combined immunodeficiency disease

This phenotype implies the presence of a defect selective to T cells for development and survival. In humans, T cells uniquely require signaling through the IL-7 and T-cell receptors during development to prevent apoptosis. The most common causes of B-positive, NK-positive SCID involve defects in these 2 signaling pathways. In terms of IL-7 signaling, it must be understood that the IL-7 receptor is composed of an α chain and γc. Although γc is shared by other cytokine receptors, IL-7Rα is not. In the United States, most cases of B-positive, NK-positive SCID occur as a result of *IL7R* (IL-7Rα) deficiency.[9,24] Rarer defects in components of the T-cell receptor have also been reported to cause SCID, including mutations in *CD3D*,[25–28] *CD3E*,[26] and *CD247*,[29,30] which encode the CD3 δ, ϵ, and ζ chains, respectively. Defects in *CD3G*[31,32] have not yet been observed to cause true SCID. In addition, CD45 (encoded by *PTPRC*) is a protein tyrosine phosphatase that is critical for regulation of T-cell receptor signaling. Several investigators have demonstrated that CD45 deficiency results in B-positive, NK-positive SCID.[33–35] Finally, defects in *CORO1A* have been shown to cause B-positive, NK-positive SCID.[36,37] The exact pathogenesis remains unknown. In mice, lack of coronin 1A impairs egress of T cells from the thymus. The protein also plays a critical role in lymphocyte F-actin dynamics, which affects homeostasis.[38] It seems likely that these 2 mechanisms work together to cause SCID.

B-negative, natural killer–negative severe combined immunodeficiency disease

This phenotype points toward a cause that affects all lymphocytes. For example, because lymphocytes proliferate, they must rapidly metabolize and synthesize DNA. ADA is necessary for degradation of deoxyadenosine triphosphate and deoxyadenosine nucleotide metabolites as part of the purine salvage pathway.[39] Purine nucleoside phosphorylase (PNP) is another critical enzyme in the purine salvage pathway that is responsible for metabolism of both deoxyadenosine and deoxyguanosine. ADA and PNP deficiency result in accumulation of purine metabolites.[39,40] These metabolic intermediates not only are toxic to lymphocytes but also directly induce apoptosis through receptor interactions, leading to B-negative, NK-negative SCID.[41–43] In another example, mitochondrial adenylate kinase 2 (AK2) regulates transfer of phosphate groups between adenine nucleotides and directly interacts with caspase-associated apoptotic pathways. Because this process also affects granulocytes, *AK2* deficiency causes a severe form of B-negative, NK-negative SCID, reticular dysgenesis, that is usually accompanied by significant neutropenia and deafness.[44,45] Separate criteria have been established for diagnosis of reticular dysgenesis.[2]

Other genetic defects have been associated with the diagnosis of SCID and are presented in **Table 2**. DNA ligase IV, Cernunnos, and PNP deficiency are not recognized as SCID causing by the International Union of Immunological Societies (IUIS) Expert Committee for Primary Immunodeficiency.[5] They are listed separately with other defects that are often designated as causes of SCID. Presentations for many of these other deficiencies, as provided in the literature, do not meet PIDTC criteria for typical SCID. In the United States, the most common cause of SCID is *IL2RG* deficiency, followed by defects in *IL7R*, *RAG1/RAG2*, *ADA*, *JAK3*, and then *DCLRE1C*.[46] In more than 30% of patients, the genetic cause remains unknown.[46]

Special considerations: T-positive severe combined immunodeficiency disease

Some infants with SCID may have detectable, normal, or even elevated numbers of circulating T cells. It has been recognized that some patients bear hypomorphic mutations in known SCID-causing genes, allowing for production of a small number of T cells.[47,48] This condition is often termed leaky SCID, although arguably the combined immunodeficiency present in these patients falls short of severe. Nonetheless, the PIDTC has established a separate stratum for these patients.[2] T cells found in untreated patients with SCID typically represent oligoclonal populations and bear CD45RO, a memory T cell phenotypic marker.[49–51] Thus, numbers and percentages of naive T cells and TREC quantities remain low. In patients with true SCID, these T cells most commonly represent either Omenn syndrome or engraftment of maternal T cells.

In 1965, Gilbert Omenn reported reticuloendotheliosis, eosinophilia, and marked susceptibility to infections in 12 male and female infants from an inbred Irish Catholic family.[52] This syndrome is now classically associated with an erythematous (often exfoliative) rash, lymphadenopathy, hepatosplenomegaly, chronic diarrhea, eosinophilia, and elevations in serum IgE and liver transaminase levels.[2,53] Omenn syndrome is thought to occur because of minimal spontaneous or residual V(D)J recombination activity that permits generation of a few T-cell clones.[50,54] The T cells are typically activated and proliferate readily. Thus, mitogen stimulation tests can yield normal or even elevated results, presenting an element of confusion for some clinicians.[53,55] The T cells do not provide protection against infections, however, and patients remain immune deficient. Children with Omenn syndrome require immune suppression to control the inflammation and damage caused by the T-cell clones. Treatment regimens may include corticosteroids and calcineurin inhibitors and lie beyond the scope of this article. Patients with B-negative, NK-positive SCID should be observed closely for development of Omenn syndrome, as it is known to occur most commonly in RAG1, RAG2, Artemis, and DNA ligase IV deficiency.[53,56] It has also appeared in other types of SCID not caused by V(D)J recombination defects, such as *IL7R* deficiency[53] and *IL2RG* deficiency.[53,55] The PIDTC has established separate criteria to help ascertain the diagnosis of Omenn syndrome.[2]

Engraftment of maternal T cells is known to transpire not infrequently in patients with SCID.[57,58] Transplacental migration of maternal T cells into the fetus occurs as a normal process during pregnancy, but the cells are typically eliminated by fetal T cells.[57,58] Thus, in patients with SCID who lack functional T cells, the transferred maternal T cells persist. These cells tend to be refractory to mitogenic stimulation.[51,58] They can be antigenically activated and mediate graft-versus-host disease (GVHD) or rejection of allogeneic hematopoietic stem cell grafts.[51,58] In a patient with SCID and T cells, maternal engraftment should be distinguished from leaky SCID or Omenn syndrome by performing tests to identify maternal T cells.[57,59]

Clinical evaluation and management

Evaluation and management of patients with SCID or suspected SCID should be performed carefully to establish the diagnosis and optimize quality of life. Clinical assessments should incorporate the medical history with laboratory testing, whereas management should focus on preventing the development of infections before definitive therapy (**Box 1**).

Clinical assessments remain key for confirming or excluding the diagnosis of SCID. In terms of medical history, patients identified through newborn screening programs may be healthy. However, late presentations may be characterized by a history of nystatin-resistant thrush or recurrent infections, particularly affecting the ears and

Box 1
Evaluation and management of patients with suspected or known SCID who have not received definitive therapy

Clinical assessments of patients with suspected SCID

Medical history

- Abnormal newborn screening test for SCID
- Recurrent or opportunistic infections

Family history

- Known primary immunodeficiency disease
- Infant deaths, especially maternal uncles

Physical examination

- Minimal tonsillar and lymph node tissue
- Signs of Omenn syndrome (lymphadenopathy, hepatosplenomegaly, and rash)
- Microcephaly

Laboratory assessments of patients with suspected SCID

- Complete blood count with manual differential to evaluate for lymphopenia
- Quantitative serum immunoglobulin levels
- Antibody titers to immunizations (if the patient is older than 6 months)
- T-cell proliferative response to phytohemagglutinin
- Enumeration of lymphocyte subsets, including naive T-cell number and percentage
- Ancillary tests as needed (serum uric acid or liver transaminase levels, TCRVβ repertoire analysis, tests for transplacentally acquired maternal T cells)
- Chest radiography to assess for a thymic shadow
- Genetic testing

Management of patients with suspected or known SCID who have not received definitive therapy

- Isolation from sources of infections, such as sick family members, day care, and hospital settings, but confinement to home is not necessary
- Universal precautions and good hand washing
- Prophylaxis against *Pneumocystis jirovecii*
- Immunoglobulin replacement therapy
- Immunizations: Live vaccines should not be administered. Household contacts should not receive oral poliovirus vaccines because of the risk for transmission to the patient. Other live vaccines may be administered to household contacts. If the vaccine recipient develops symptoms of infection, contact with the patient should be avoided
- Aggressive treatment of infections: Infections should be recognized promptly, and unusual pathogens should be considered. Antibiotic therapy should be started early and discontinued cautiously
- Transfusion of only irradiated, cytomegalovirus-negative, leukocyte-depleted blood products when needed
- Immune suppression for patients with suspected or known Omenn syndrome
- Avoidance of ionizing radiation in patients with suspected or known B-negative, NK-positive SCID, when possible

lungs. It remains vital to obtain a family history centered on questions regarding consanguinity and recurrent infections or infant deaths (or known primary immunodeficiency disease). For suspected *IL2RG* deficiency in a male infant, early mortality of any maternal uncles should be noted. Physical examination remains important: patients with SCID have minimal tonsillar and lymph node tissue, whereas lymphadenopathy and hepatosplenomegaly with rash may be present in a patient with Omenn syndrome. Microcephaly may point toward DNA ligase IV or Cernunnos deficiency. Next, laboratory testing is needed to confirm or exclude the diagnosis. A complete blood count with manual differential should be performed, as almost all patients with typical SCID have absolute lymphocyte counts less than 2,000 cells/mm^3.[60] Quantitative serum immunoglobulin levels are low in patients with SCID with the exception of maternally transferred IgG that is present during infancy. Because of this IgG, testing for specific antibody function is generally not helpful until after 6 months of age. One key test that must be performed as immediately as possible is assessment of the T-cell response to PHA. Testing for proliferation to antigens, such as *Candida* or tetanus, is not necessary to confirm or exclude the diagnosis of SCID. Enumeration of lymphocyte subsets represents the other essential test that should be performed with highest priority. The test is critical for not only determining the T-cell count but also for classifying the patient by B-cell and NK-cell status until a genetic diagnosis can eventually be made. Evaluation of naive T-cell counts and numbers is no longer required, especially because various laboratories use inconsistent means to differentiate CD45RA$^+$ T cells. Ancillary laboratory tests may provide helpful information. If PNP deficiency is suspected, a low serum uric acid may provide support for the diagnosis. Patients with Omenn syndrome should have liver transaminase levels monitored. TCRVβ repertoire testing can be performed if T cells are present and the provider feels the need to confirm oligoclonality. To identify maternal T cells, short tandem repeat or variable number tandem repeat testing of isolated T cells should be performed. Chest radiographs in infants may support the diagnosis of SCID if a thymic shadow is absent. Patients with *CORO1A* deficiency, however, can have a normal thymic appearance radiographically. Finally, genetic testing should be performed (see **Table 1**), although lack of genetic diagnosis should not preclude definitive therapy.

Management of patients with SCID or suspected SCID should emphasize awareness of the profound T- and B-cell defects. Infants should be kept isolated from household members with infections as much as possible. It is also recommended that they be kept in reverse isolation with respiratory and contact precautions in hospital settings. The family must be taught universal precautions and strict handwashing techniques. The untreated patient should avoid social gatherings, if possible, but excursions from the house for necessary activities should not be harmful. The risk for infection in all of these settings must be minimized by initiating prophylaxis against *Pneumocystis jirovecii* and immunoglobulin replacement therapy. Candidal prophylaxis may be considered as well but is not uniformly practiced. Except for live polio virus (no longer available in the United States), all household members should be kept immunized, but the patient should not receive any live viral or bacterial immunizations.[61] Any acute infections must be treated aggressively, and providers should set a low threshold for hospital admission. If transfusion of blood products is needed, they must be leukocyte reduced, irradiated, and cytomegalovirus negative. Patients with Omenn syndrome should be treated with immune suppression, as discussed earlier. Finally, patients who have DNA repair defects must be identified quickly because failure to repair DNA damage can increase the risk for future malignancy. The patients are radiosensitive[62] and should minimize exposure to sunlight, ultraviolet light, and ionizing radiation, such as gamma radiation delivered during radiologic studies. Thus, it would be reasonable to minimize these exposures in patients with B-negative, NK-positive SCID until a genetic diagnosis can be confirmed. In addition, providers who perform hematopoietic stem cell transplant must be made aware of increased sensitivity of tissues to DNA cross-linking medications and adjust any conditioning regimens accordingly.[62,63] For example, use of alkylator therapy in Artemis deficiency should be avoided because it is associated with poor growth, abnormal dental development, and late endocrinopathies.[64] In summary, although patients with SCID do not need to be treated delicately, they should be managed closely and carefully. Children with SCID who have become fully immunoreconstituted through hematopoietic stem cell transplant or gene therapy should attend regular school to develop the social and educational skills essential for their development as a person and their integration into society.

Treatment

History

In 1971, a boy was born in Houston, Texas. His parents had previously given birth to another boy, who had died at 7 months of age because of SCID. The mother was suspected to carry an unknown SCID-causing gene in one of her X chromosomes, and this newborn boy was therefore placed in sterile containment immediately after birth. The infant was indeed fully deficient in T- and B-cell function,[65] and the older sister was determined to be HLA-nonidentical. For lack of any other curative therapies at that time, the boy was kept in a plastic, germ-free chamber. He became known to the world as David the Bubble Boy. David grew and learned to interact with physicians and family members outside of the chamber (**Fig. 1**). In 1977, NASA researchers even developed a specialized suit that would enable him to walk for short distances outside of the chamber while remaining in complete isolation. David lived until the age of 12 years, when he died of Epstein-Barr virus (EBV) infection after T-cell-depleted mismatched related donor hematopoietic bone marrow stem cell transplant.[66] Nearly 10 years later, investigators identified his genetic defect in one of the groundbreaking publications that demonstrated *IL2RG* deficiency as the cause of X-linked SCID.[3] Today, SCID is sometimes still referred to as the bubble boy disease. At the time, David was the longest known survivor of the condition. Now, therapeutic options have improved substantially, and definitive cure is possible.

Two forms of definitive therapy are available: hematopoietic bone marrow stem cell transplant and gene therapy. Polyethylene glycol-conjugated adenosine deaminase (PEG-ADA) infusions may provide a third option for patients with ADA deficiency,[67–69] but PEG-ADA treatment is no longer favored because it does not permanently correct the defect, and immunologic deficiencies persist despite enzyme therapy.[70] Stem cell transplant for primary immunodeficiency diseases is discussed in detail by Hagin D and colleagues,[71] so the summary here lightly mentions transplant approaches and focuses on unresolved issues and long-term outcomes. Gene therapy is offered only in clinical research trials but is nonetheless reviewed because it will likely become widely available in the future.

Hematopoietic bone marrow stem cell transplant

The first successful hematopoietic stem cell transplant using bone marrow from a non-twin relative to treat SCID or any other disease was performed in 1968 by Dr Robert A. Good in a boy with X-linked SCID.[72,73] The donor was an older sister, who was HLA-identical. Most patients did not have an HLA-identical sibling donor and remained untreated. In 1973, successful stem cell transplant for SCID using bone marrow

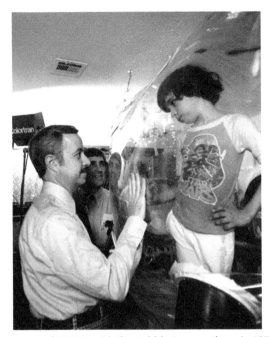

Fig. 1. Early management of SCID. David, the Bubble Boy, was born in 1971 with SCID due to *IL2RG* deficiency. Hematopoietic bone marrow stem cell transplant was not possible at that time in the absence of an HLA-identical sibling donor. David is shown within his plastic, pathogen-free chamber at Texas Children's Hospital in Houston, Texas, holding his hand up to the hand of Dr William T. Shearer, his physician. (*From* Shearer WT, Demaret CA. David's story. In: Etzioni A, Ochs H, editors. Primary immunodeficiency disorders: a historic and scientific perspective. Philadelphia: Elsevier; 2014. p. 323; with permission.)

from an unrelated donor was reported, but the donor did not show mixed lymphocyte culture reactivity toward the recipient, suggesting a high degree of HLA identity.[74] The first successful stem cell transplant for SCID using bone marrow from a truly HLA-mismatched donor was published in 1977 and used a cyclophosphamide conditioning regimen.[75] Soon afterward, successful hematopoietic stem cell transplant for leukemia was demonstrated using donor bone marrow that had been treated with soybean lectin and sheep erythrocytes.[76] For SCID, it was revealed in 1983 that the same protocol could be used to rigorously deplete T cells from donor bone marrow and allow for successful haploidentical hematopoietic stem cell transplant without conditioning.[77] Thus, all patients with SCID could receive parental bone marrow stem cell transplant. Since then, various protocols have been developed for hematopoietic stem cell transplant in patients with SCID involving identical, parental, and HLA-matched unrelated donors both with and without conditioning. As a result, many controversial issues exist regarding optimal transplant methods.[63,78]

The most controversial issue surrounds the use or absence of conditioning for haploidentical or HLA-matched unrelated donor transplant in terms of effects on B-cell function, NK-cell function, and late complications. In terms of B cells, reconstitution using parental donor bone marrow cells without conditioning (but with rigorous T-cell depletion) has been reported, but efficacy varies by molecular defect.[79,80] With this protocol, B-cell donor chimerism is rarely achieved (greatest for *IL2RG* and *ADA* deficiency at 36% and 33%, respectively). About half of survivors continue to require immunoglobulin replacement, 62% of whom have *IL2RG* deficiency, for which B-cell reconstitution is known to be challenging.[12] More than 80% of patients with *RAG1* and *RAG2* deficiency also continue to require immunoglobulin replacement therapy. However, patients with *IL7R* (94%), *ADA* (78%), and CD3 component deficiencies (100%) develop normal B-cell function and are able to discontinue immunoglobulin infusions. These data suggest that donor chimerism is dispensable, and hence conditioning is not needed, for B-cell function in patients who have molecular defects that do not affect B-cell activity. On the other hand, conditioning may be helpful for patients who require donor B-cell chimerism due to intrinsic recipient B-cell defects (eg, *IL2RG*, *JAK3*, *RAG1*, *RAG2*, and *DCLRE1C* deficiency). For HLA-matched unrelated donor transplant without conditioning in patients with SCID,[81] T-cell engraftment occurs in similar degree to HLA-matched sibling donor transplant, but risk for GVHD is increased, and B-cell reconstitution is impaired.[82] Regarding NK cells, some investigators have argued that conditioning is needed to remove NK cells that may oppose donor T- and B-cell engraftment, such as in *RAG1* and *RAG2* deficiency.[83] Other researchers have disputed that assertion.[84] Thus, the issue remains unresolved. Disseminated cutaneous human papillomavirus infections have been reported after hematopoietic stem cell transplant in patients with *IL2RG* and *JAK3* deficiency, suggesting that donor NK-cell engraftment should be encouraged in these 2 conditions.[85,86] Finally, in terms of late effects, complications vary depending on use or absence of conditioning. With the use of conditioning, problems after 2 years posttransplant include death from GVHD (7%), chronic GVHD (10%), secondary malignancies and lymphoproliferative disease (2%–3%), need for long-term nutritional support (20%), human papillomavirus infections (25%), autoimmune or inflammatory complications (13%), and cognitive difficulties.[63] The risk for neuropsychiatric problems after use of chemotherapeutic agents remains acknowledged[87,88] and closely observed with recognition of the fact that ADA-,[89] Cernunnos-, and DNA ligase IV–deficient patients develop neurocognitive deficits because the molecular defects affect central nervous system tissues in manners that cannot be corrected by hematopoietic stem cell transplant. With use of rigorous T-cell depletion and no conditioning, late effects include minimal (<5%) prevalence of cutaneous GVHD, autoimmune disease, thyroid disease, seizure disorder, and cerebral palsy.[90,91] Diarrhea (15%) and human papillomavirus infections (10%) are observed. Developmental delay is reported in less than 10% of patients, whereas attention-deficit hyperactivity disorder is noted in approximately 20%. Much of the data concerning use of conditioning come from Europe, where V(D)J recombination defects and autosomal recessive forms of SCID occur more frequently than observed in the United States. Thus, data for use and absence of conditioning within the United States would provide better comparisons.

In 2014, the PIDTC published these data in a summary of outcomes of hematopoietic stem cell transplant for SCID performed in 25 centers in the United States from 2000 to 2009.[46] Overall, the results indicate that use of matched sibling donors yields the best outcomes. A previous study had shown superior T-cell reconstitution and improved survival if transplant is performed before 3.5 months of age.[92] The PIDTC findings supported these observations, including a survival rate of 94% for infants who underwent transplant before 3.5 months of age regardless of use or absence of conditioning. This enhanced survival correlated strongly with absence of infection before or at the time of transplant. For actively infected infants, optimal survival was achieved using matched sibling donors, but haploidentical transplant without conditioning presented the next best survival. Overall, use of conditioning was associated with greater likelihood for developing higher T-cell counts and clinically relevant B-cell function but correlated significantly with decreased survival. Thus, use of conditioning may be considered if the family desires a higher chance for discontinuing immunoglobulin replacement therapy after transplant and the patient is younger than 3.5 months, but conditioning should almost certainly be avoided in patients with active infections. Use of conditioning to modulate NK-cell function and late sequelae after conditioning remain unaddressed by the PIDTC.

Gene therapy

Gene therapy trials were initiated to treat *ADA* and *IL2RG* deficiency in 1990 and 1999, respectively. Onset of the trial for *ADA* deficiency marked the first ever attempted use of gene therapy to correct a human disease. Gene therapy for *ADA* deficiency has demonstrated marked success in all trials to date.[93-96] For *IL2RG*, although 18 of the initial 20 recipients of gene therapy showed successful immune reconstitution, 5 developed leukemia due to insertional mutagenesis of the retroviral vector within the *LMO2* oncogene.[97-99] No similar leukemia or insertional mutagenesis has been observed in any of the *ADA* deficiency gene therapy trials.[100-102] Subsequently, all gene therapy trials for *IL2RG* deficiency were halted. Before the trials were halted, researchers found that gene therapy for *IL2RG* deficiency does not work well in older patients, suggesting an optimal window of time to conduct the procedure.[103] Investigators raced to find a new vector and ultimately focused on a self-inactivating γ-retrovirus vector. In 2010, gene therapy for *IL2RG* deficiency was restarted using this vector.[104] A total of 9 patients were treated with 8 survivors. With 1 to 3 years of follow-up, no insertional mutagenesis has been detected. The survivors have demonstrated appropriate gene marking in T cells and immune reconstitution. Other investigators are beginning to develop lentiviral vectors[105] with self-inactivating capability.[106] Thus, additional clinical trials are anticipated soon. Overall, gene therapy trials for SCID have shown significant promise as a treatment strategy that is expected to become more widely available if eventually approved by the Food and Drug Administration (FDA) for use in the United States.

Congenital Athymia

Diagnostic considerations

Lack of sufficient thymic function also produces a severe combined T-negative, B-positive, NK-positive immune deficiency that meets PIDTC criteria for typical SCID yet is associated with complete DiGeorge anomaly or *FOXN1* deficiency. DiGeorge anomaly is characterized by defects of the heart, thymus, and parathyroid glands that may occur to varying degrees.[107-111] Despite the widely used practice of excluding the diagnosis based on testing for 22q11.2 hemizygosity, the diagnosis is established clinically. Less than 60%[112-114] of patients with DiGeorge anomaly have 22q11.2 hemizygosity, indicating that some patients are missed or inappropriately treated if only 22q11.2 deletions are considered. Other known causes of DiGeorge anomaly include CHARGE (ie, *c*oloboma, *h*eart defect, *a*tresia or stenosis of the choanae, *r*etardation of development or growth, *g*enitourinary abnormality, *e*ar malformation) syndrome (which is often but not always associated with *CHD7* defects), VACTERL (ie, *v*ertebral abnormality, *a*nal atresia, *c*ardiac defect, *t*racheoesophageal anomaly, *r*enal or radial defect, *l*imb malformation) association, and diabetic embryopathy.[112-114] Thus, genetic testing cannot be used to exclude the diagnosis. In as many as 2% of patients with DiGeorge anomaly,[115] congenital athymia is present, resulting in the diagnosis of complete DiGeorge anomaly. Partial DiGeorge anomaly is characterized by some degree of thymic function and remains 50 times more prevalent. In terms of *FOXN1* deficiency, the phenotype was first reported in animal models in the 1960s, consisting of alopecia totalis and athymia.[116,117] In the 1990s, the genetic cause was identified in animal models[118] and in humans.[119,120]

FOXN1 encodes a winged-helix/forkhead protein needed for differentiation of certain epithelial cells, in particular thymic epithelium. Thus, *FOXN1* deficiency produces the observed clinical phenotype.

The diagnosis of congenital athymia is traditionally established by the presence of fewer than 50 naive T cells/mm^3 in peripheral blood or less than 5% of total T cells in the circulation having a naive phenotype.[114,121,122] In all infants who exhibit any clinical features of DiGeorge anomaly, it remains essential to use these criteria to distinguish complete DiGeorge anomaly from partial DiGeorge anomaly. Patients with athymia lack T-cell responses to PHA and fail to produce protective antibodies, resulting in a severe combined T- and B-cell deficiency that results in death from infection by 2 years of age if left untreated.[113,121] Some infants (more than 40% for complete DiGeorge anomaly[114]) progress from typical athymia to an atypical presentation that closely resembles Omenn syndrome.[123,124] Findings include erythrodermic rash, lymphadenopathy, hepatosplenomegaly, and elevated serum liver transaminase levels and are associated with the presence of activated, oligoclonal expansions of T cells that can exhibit normal or enhanced proliferation to PHA.[113,114,123,124] These infants ultimately require immunosuppression using corticosteroids and calcineurin inhibitors to minimize systemic damage from the T cells.[113,125] For long-term survival, all patients with congenital athymia require definitive therapy.

Treatment strategies
Two options are available to promote long-term survival. Allogeneic thymus transplant presents the first option but is provided with limited availability because of restrictions from the FDA, which designates it as a research method. It will be provocative to observe the ramifications of this limited availability as identification of congenital athymia accelerates in the United States due to increased newborn screening for SCID. The other option involves the use of bone marrow transplant or mature T-cell infusions. This method provides T cells, but recipients remain unable to generate naive T cells. Thus, each method has its disadvantages.

Thymus transplant
Allogeneic thymus transplant has demonstrated significant success for treatment of congenital athymia. The process involves the use of discarded thymus tissue, with informed consent, from an HLA-non-matched infant younger than 9 months who is undergoing cardiac surgery.[113] The thymus tissue is transected and cultured for up to 3 weeks while donor screening is performed according to FDA regulations.[113] The tissue is then surgically embedded within the recipient's quadriceps muscles. After 6 to 12 months, recipients develop a broad repertoire of naive[113,125] and regulatory[126] T cells. Normal T-cell proliferation to PHA and tetanus is observed and accompanied by the ability to discontinue immunoglobulin replacement therapy, but T-cell counts remain low.[113,122,125,127] For patients who develop the atypical presentation, thymus transplant results in disappearance of T-cell-mediated inflammatory disease and ability to discontinue immune suppression.[113,122–126] Pretransplant infections resolve.[113,122,125] Despite lack of HLA matching between donors and recipients and absence of GVHD prophylaxis, no GVHD is observed, perhaps due to depletion of donor thymocytes during the thymus graft culturing process.[113] Recipients develop tolerance toward the grafts and third-party tissues HLA matched to the grafts.[128,129] Allogeneic thymus transplant results in overall survival of 73%[113,122,125] (100% for *FOXN1* deficiency[113]). In terms of long-term sequelae, approximately one-third of patients develop autoimmune thyroid disease for reasons that remain unclear.[113] It is not

known whether thymus transplant is able to correct the functional NK-cell deficiency that is known to occur in some patients with 22q11.2 hemizygosity.[130]

Bone marrow transplant or mature T-cell infusions

Complete DiGeorge anomaly and FOXN1 deficiency have both been treated using either hematopoietic bone marrow stem cell transplant or mature T-cell infusions from HLA-matched siblings, matched unrelated donors, or a parent.[131–137] For complete DiGeorge anomaly, a review of 17 treated patients demonstrated 41% overall survival.[136] Although patients develop normal T cell numbers through clonal expansion and normal proliferative responses to PHA, a significant issue that remains unaddressed involves persistent lack of thymic function. This problem precludes the ability for recipients to generate T cells against novel pathogens not encountered by the donor, such as EBV.[113,132,138] Thus, transplant of bone marrow or mature T cells does not provide the most preferred option for treatment of congenital athymia.

Newborn Screening for Severe Combined Immunodeficiency Disorders

Implementation and outcomes

Newborn screening has been established in the United States as an effective method to identify patients with SCID and other forms of T-cell lymphopenia, such as congenital athymia. Because patients with SCID demonstrate absence of recent thymic emigrants, a test was developed to identify low TREC counts in Guthrie card blood spots.[139] TRECs do not replicate when T cells divide, so counts remain low even in patients with SCID who have clonally expanded T cells. This test now serves as the basis for all newborn screening tests for SCID in the United States. The screening programs are calculated to yield financial benefits over time in terms of reducing health care costs,[140,141] and early identification of affected infants permits transplant before the critical threshold of age 3.5 months[46,80] for optimal immune reconstitution and survival. Statewide newborn screening was first implemented in Wisconsin in 2008.[142] Since then, approximately half of the 50 states have begun screening. The outcomes of screening in 11 of these states have been reported.[143] The results demonstrate that newborn screening identified 52 infants with typical SCID, leaky SCID, or Omenn syndrome of about 3 million tests performed. These initial figures have established the incidence of SCID at 1 per 58,000 live births (and 1 per 72,000 live births for typical SCID alone).[143] Of the 52 identified infants, 49 were able to receive immune-restoring therapies, and long-term survival has been demonstrated in 92% of these treated children.[143] Thus, the programs have yielded significant success.

Considerations

With broad implementation of newborn screening for SCID, 2 issues have come to the forefront. First, providers have become increasingly faced with management decisions concerning infants with idiopathic T-cell lymphopenia.[143] These infants have persistently low numbers of T cells and immune dysfunction yet do not possess defects in known SCID genes or meet PIDTC criteria for SCID.[143] Approximately 1 of every 250,000 infants screened has idiopathic T-cell lymphopenia.[143] Close observation is recommended (1 patient has required hematopoietic stem cell transplant) but consensus has not been reached regarding optimal management strategies.[143] This issue will likely need to be addressed in the near future. Second, clinicians are being challenged to distinguish between SCID and congenital athymia, especially when 22q11.2 hemizygosity or *CHD7* mutations are not present. To confuse matters further, SCID can be present in children with 22q11.2 deletions.[144] Proper diagnosis remains essential because children with SCID should not be given thymus transplant, and hematopoietic bone marrow stem cell transplant may not provide the optimal solution for congenital athymia. It has been established that the newborn screening test for SCID readily identifies children with DiGeorge anomaly.[115,145] In the United States, approximately 1 of every 37,000 infants tested has 22q11.2 hemizygosity or CHARGE syndrome with T-cell lymphopenia significant enough to be captured by the newborn screening test.[143] Three infants with abnormal newborn screening results have been diagnosed with complete DiGeorge anomaly.[143] Thus, providers must begin to learn and develop strategies to distinguish complete DiGeorge anomaly (eg, presence of hypoparathyroidism, cardiac defects, or other anatomic abnormalities or history of diabetic embryopathy) and *FOXN1* deficiency (eg, absence of hair) from SCID in the presence of negative genetic testing results.

FUTURE CONSIDERATIONS/SUMMARY

During the last 4 to 5 decades, the medical and scientific communities have come far in recognizing how to identify, manage, and treat patients born with severe combined immunodeficiency disorders. With improved understanding of the cellular and molecular causes of congenital T-cell deficiencies, attention now necessarily shifts toward optimizing strategies to minimize long-term mortality and morbidity in patients who are treated. With widespread implementation of newborn screening programs for these conditions, novel challenges are anticipated to appear, which must be embraced and resolved. Thus, although the substantial accomplishments by so many people to date deserve much celebration, efforts must continue until all patients can be given the best possible outcomes.

REFERENCES

1. Griffith LM, Cowan MJ, Notarangelo LD, et al. Improving cellular therapy for primary immune deficiency diseases: recognition, diagnosis, and management. J Allergy Clin Immunol 2009;124:1152–60.e12.
2. Shearer WT, Dunn E, Notarangelo LD, et al. Establishing diagnostic criteria for severe combined immunodeficiency disease (SCID), leaky SCID, and Omenn syndrome: the Primary Immune Deficiency Treatment Consortium experience. J Allergy Clin Immunol 2014;133:1092–8.
3. Noguchi M, Yi H, Rosenblatt HM, et al. Interleukin-2 receptor γ chain mutation results in X-linked severe combined immunodeficiency in humans. Cell 1993; 73:147–57.
4. Puck JM, Deschenes SM, Porter JC, et al. The interleukin-2 receptor γ chain maps to Xq13.1 and is mutated in X-linked severe combined immunodeficiency, SCIDX1. Hum Mol Genet 1993;2:1099–104.
5. Al-Herz W, Bousfiha A, Casanova J-L, et al. Primary immunodeficiency diseases: an update on the classification from the International Union Of Immunological Societies Expert Committee for primary immunodeficiency. Front Immunol 2014;5:162.
6. Nijman IJ, van Montfrans JM, Hoogstraat M, et al. Targeted next-generation sequencing: a novel diagnostic tool for primary immunodeficiencies. J Allergy Clin Immunol 2014;133:529–34.e1.
7. Kohn LA, Seet CS, Scholes J, et al. Human lymphoid development in the absence of common γ-chain receptor signaling. J Immunol 2014;192(11): 5050–8.
8. Kovanen PE, Leonard WJ. Cytokines and immunodeficiency diseases: critical roles of the γc-dependent cytokines interleukins 2, 4, 7, 9, 15, and 21, and their signaling pathways. Immunol Rev 2004;202:67–83.

9. Roifman CM, Zhang J, Chitayat D, et al. A partial deficiency of interleukin-7Rα is sufficient to abrogate T-cell development and cause severe combined immunodeficiency. Blood 2000;96:2803–7.

10. Vosshenrich CAJ, Ranson T, Samson SI, et al. Roles for common cytokine receptor γ-chain-dependent cytokines in the generation, differentiation, and maturation of NK cell precursors and peripheral NK Cells in vivo. J Immunol 2005;174:1213–21.

11. Meazza R, Azzarone B, Orengo AM, et al. Role of common-gamma chain cytokines in NK cell development and function: perspectives for immunotherapy. J Biomed Biotechnol 2011;2011:861920.

12. White H, Thrasher A, Veys P, et al. Intrinsic defects of B cell function in X-linked severe combined immunodeficiency. Eur J Immunol 2000;30:732–7.

13. Buckley RH. Molecular defects in human severe combined immunodeficiency and approaches to immune reconstitution. Annu Rev Immunol 2004;22:625–55.

14. Cacalano NA, Migone TS, Bazan F, et al. Autosomal SCID caused by a point mutation in the N-terminus of Jak3: mapping of the Jak3–receptor interaction domain. EMBO J 1999;18:1549–58.

15. Macchi P, Villa A, Giliani S, et al. Mutations of Jak-3 gene in patients with autosomal severe combined immune deficiency (SCID). Nature 1995;377:65–8.

16. Li L, Moshous D, Zhou Y, et al. A founder mutation in artemis, an SNM1-like protein, causes SCID in Athabascan-speaking Native Americans. J Immunol 2002; 168:6323–9.

17. Moshous D, Callebaut I, de Chasseval R, et al. Artemis, a novel DNA double-strand break repair/V(D)J recombination protein, is mutated in human severe combined immune deficiency. Cell 2001;105:177–86.

18. Nicolas N, Moshous D, Cavazzana-Calvo M, et al. A human severe combined immunodeficiency (SCID) condition with increased sensitivity to ionizing radiations and impaired V(D)J rearrangements defines a new DNA recombination/repair deficiency. J Exp Med 1998;188:627–34.

19. van der Burg M, Ijspeert H, Verkaik NS, et al. A DNA-PKcs mutation in a radiosensitive T(–)B(–) SCID patient inhibits Artemis activation and nonhomologous end-joining. J Clin Invest 2009;119:91–8.

20. van der Burg M, van Veelen LR, Verkaik NS, et al. A new type of radiosensitive T–B–NK+ severe combined immunodeficiency caused by a LIG4 mutation. J Clin Invest 2006;116:137–45.

21. Enders A, Fisch P, Schwarz K, et al. A severe form of human combined immunodeficiency due to mutations in DNA Ligase IV. J Immunol 2006;176:5060–8.

22. Buck D, Moshous D, de Chasseval R, et al. Severe combined immunodeficiency and microcephaly in siblings with hypomorphic mutations in DNA ligase IV. Eur J Immunol 2006;36:224–35.

23. Buck D, Malivert L, de Chasseval R, et al. Cernunnos, a novel nonhomologous end-joining factor, is mutated in human immunodeficiency with microcephaly. Cell 2006;124:287–99.

24. Puel A, Ziegler SF, Buckley RH, et al. Defective IL7R expression in T-B+NK+ severe combined immunodeficiency. Nat Genet 1998;20:394–7.

25. Siegers GM, Swamy M, Fernández-Malavé E, et al. Different composition of the human and the mouse γδ T cell receptor explains different phenotypes of CD3γ and CD3δ immunodeficiencies. J Exp Med 2007;204:2537–44.

26. de Saint Basile G, Geissmann F, Flori E, et al. Severe combined immunodeficiency caused by deficiency in either the δ or the ε subunit of CD3. J Clin Invest 2004;114:1512–7.

27. Dadi HK, Simon AJ, Roifman CM. Effect of CD3δ deficiency on maturation of α/β and γ/δ T-cell lineages in severe combined immunodeficiency. N Engl J Med 2003;349:1821–8.
28. Gil J, Busto EM, Garcillán B, et al. A leaky mutation in CD3D differentially affects αβ and γδ T cells and leads to a Tαβ(−)Tγδ(+)B(+)NK(+) human SCID. J Clin Invest 2011;121:3872–6.
29. Rieux-Laucat F, Hivroz C, Lim A, et al. Inherited and somatic CD3ζ mutations in a patient with T-cell deficiency. N Engl J Med 2006;354:1913–21.
30. Roberts JL, Lauritsen JPH, Cooney M, et al. T(−)B(+)NK(+) severe combined immunodeficiency caused by complete deficiency of the CD3ζ subunit of the T-cell antigen receptor complex. Blood 2007;109:3198–206.
31. Arnaiz-Villena A, Timon M, Rodriguez-Gallego C, et al. T lymphocyte signalling defects and immunodeficiency due to the lack of CD3 gamma. Immunodeficiency 1993;4:121–9.
32. Arnaiz-Villena A, Timon M, Corell A, et al. Primary immunodeficiency caused by mutations in the gene encoding the CD3-γ subunit of the T-lymphocyte receptor. N Engl J Med 1992;327:529–33.
33. Tchilian EZ, Wallace DL, Wells RS, et al. A deletion in the gene encoding the CD45 antigen in a patient with SCID. J Immunol 2001;166:1308–13.
34. Kung C, Pingel JT, Heikinheimo M, et al. Mutations in the tyrosine phosphatase CD45 gene in a child with severe combined immunodeficiency disease. Nat Med 2000;6:343–5.
35. Roberts JL, Buckley RH, Luo B, et al. CD45-deficient severe combined immunodeficiency caused by uniparental disomy. Proc Natl Acad Sci U S A 2012;109:10456–61.
36. Shiow LR, Roadcap DW, Paris K, et al. The actin regulator coronin 1A is mutant in a thymic egress-deficient mouse strain and in a patient with severe combined immunodeficiency. Nat Immunol 2008;9:1307–15.
37. Shiow LR, Paris K, Akana MC, et al. Severe combined immunodeficiency (SCID) and attention deficit hyperactivity disorder (ADHD) associated with a coronin-1A mutation and a chromosome 16p11.2 deletion. Clin Immunol 2009;131:24–30.
38. Föger N, Rangell L, Danilenko DM, et al. Requirement for coronin 1 in T lymphocyte trafficking and cellular homeostasis. Science 2006;313:839–42.
39. Benke PJ, Dittmar D. Purine dysfunction in cells from patients with adenosine deaminase deficiency. Pediatr Res 1976;10:642–6.
40. Cohen A, Doyle D, Martin DW, et al. Abnormal purine metabolism and purine overproduction in a patient deficient in purine nucleoside phosphorylase. N Engl J Med 1976;295:1449–54.
41. Kameoka J, Tanaka T, Nojima Y, et al. Direct association of adenosine deaminase with a T cell activation antigen, CD26. Science 1993;261:466–9.
42. Markert ML. Purine nucleoside phosphorylase deficiency. Immunodefic Rev 1991;3:45–81.
43. Pannicke U, Tuchschmid P, Friedrich W, et al. Two novel missense and frameshift mutations in exons 5 and 6 of the purine nucleoside phosphorylase (PNP) gene in a severe combined immunodeficiency (SCID) patient. Hum Genet 1996;98:706–9.
44. Lagresle-Peyrou C, Six EM, Picard C, et al. Human adenylate kinase 2 deficiency causes a profound hematopoietic defect associated with sensorineural deafness. Nat Genet 2009;41:106–11.

45. Pannicke U, Honig M, Hess I, et al. Reticular dysgenesis (aleukocytosis) is caused by mutations in the gene encoding mitochondrial adenylate kinase 2. Nat Genet 2009;41:101–5.

46. Pai S-Y, Logan BR, Griffith LM, et al. Transplantation outcomes for severe combined immunodeficiency, 2000–2009. N Engl J Med 2014;371:434–46.

47. DiSanto JP, Rieux-Laucat F, Dautry-Varsat A, et al. Defective human interleukin 2 receptor gamma chain in an atypical X chromosome-linked severe combined immunodeficiency with peripheral T cells. Proc Natl Acad Sci U S A 1994;91:9466–70.

48. Schmalstieg FC, Leonard WJ, Noguchi M, et al. Missense mutation in exon 7 of the common gamma chain gene causes a moderate form of X-linked combined immunodeficiency. J Clin Invest 1995;95:1169–73.

49. Wada T, Toma T, Okamoto H, et al. Oligoclonal expansion of T lymphocytes with multiple second-site mutations leads to Omenn syndrome in a patient with RAG1-deficient severe combined immunodeficiency. Blood 2005;106: 2099–101.

50. de Saint-Basile G, Le Deist F, de Villartay JP, et al. Restricted heterogeneity of T lymphocytes in combined immunodeficiency with hypereosinophilia (Omenn's syndrome). J Clin Invest 1991;87:1352–9.

51. Palmer K, Green TD, Roberts JL, et al. Unusual clinical and immunologic manifestations of transplacentally acquired maternal T cells in severe combined immunodeficiency. J Allergy Clin Immunol 2007;120:423–8.

52. Omenn GS. Familial reticuloendotheliosis with eosinophilia. N Engl J Med 1965; 273:427–32.

53. Villa A, Notarangelo LD, Roifman CM. Omenn syndrome: inflammation in leaky severe combined immunodeficiency. J Allergy Clin Immunol 2008;122:1082–6.

54. Villa A, Santagata S, Bozzi F, et al. Partial V(D)J recombination activity leads to Omenn syndrome. Cell 1998;93:885–96.

55. Gruber TA, Shah AJ, Hernandez M, et al. Clinical and genetic heterogeneity in Omenn syndrome and severe combined immune deficiency. Pediatr Transplant 2009;13:244–50.

56. Grunebaum E, Bates A, Roifman CM. Omenn syndrome is associated with mutations in DNA ligase IV. J Allergy Clin Immunol 2008;122:1219–20.

57. Pollack MS, Kirkpatrick D, Kapoor N, et al. Identification by HLA typing of intrauterine-derived maternal T cells in four patients with severe combined immunodeficiency. N Engl J Med 1982;307:662–6.

58. Müller SM, Ege M, Pottharst A, et al. Transplacentally acquired maternal T lymphocytes in severe combined immunodeficiency: a study of 121 patients. Blood 2001;98:1847–51.

59. Appleton A, Curtis A, Wilkes J, et al. Differentiation of materno-fetal GVHD from Omenn's syndrome in pre-BMT patients with severe combined immunodeficiency. Bone Marrow Transplant 1994;14:157–9.

60. Buckley RH. The long quest for neonatal screening for severe combined immunodeficiency. J Allergy Clin Immunol 2012;129:597–604.

61. Shearer WT, Fleisher TA, Buckley RH, et al. Recommendations for live viral and bacterial vaccines in immunodeficient patients and their close contacts. J Allergy Clin Immunol 2014;133:961–6.

62. Dvorak CC, Cowan MJ. Radiosensitive severe combined immunodeficiency disease. Immunol Allergy Clin North Am 2010;30:125–42.

63. Horn B, Cowan MJ. Unresolved issues in hematopoietic stem cell transplantation for severe combined immunodeficiency: need for safer conditioning and reduced late effects. J Allergy Clin Immunol 2013;131:1306–11.

64. Schuetz C, Neven B, Dvorak CC, et al. SCID patients with ARTEMIS vs RAG deficiencies following HCT: increased risk of late toxicity in ARTEMIS-deficient SCID. Blood 2013;123:281–9.
65. South MA, Montgomery JR, Richie E, et al. Four-year study of a boy with combined immune deficiency maintained in strict reverse isolation from birth. IV. Immunologic studies. Pediatr Res 1977;11:71–8.
66. Shearer WT, Ritz J, Finegold MJ, et al. Epstein–Barr virus–associated B-cell proliferations of diverse clonal origins after bone marrow transplantation in a 12-year-old patient with severe combined immunodeficiency. N Engl J Med 1985;312:1151–9.
67. Hershfield M. Enzyme replacement therapy of adenosine deaminase deficiency with polyethylene glycol-modified adenosine deaminase (PEG-ADA). Immunodeficiency 1993;4:93–7.
68. Gaspar H. Bone marrow transplantation and alternatives for adenosine deaminase deficiency. Immunol Allergy Clin North Am 2010;30:221–36.
69. Hershfield M. PEG-ADA: an alternative to haploidentical bone marrow transplantation and an adjunct to gene therapy for adenosine deaminase deficiency. Hum Mutat 1995;5:107–12.
70. Malacarne F, Benicchi T, Notarangelo LD, et al. Reduced thymic output, increased spontaneous apoptosis and oligoclonal B cells in polyethylene glycol-adenosine deaminase-treated patients. Eur J Immunol 2005;35:3376–86.
71. Hagin D, Burroughs L, Torgerson TR. Hematopoietic Stem Cell Transplant for Immune Deficiency and Immune Dysregulation Disorders. Immunol Allergy Clin North Am 2015, in press.
72. Gatti RA, Meuwissen HJ, Allen HD, et al. Immunological reconstitution of sex-linked lymphopenic immunological deficiency. Lancet 1968;292:1366–9.
73. Meuwissen HJ, Gatti RA, Terasaki PI, et al. Treatment of lymphopenic hypogammaglobulinemia and bone-marrow aplasia by transplantation of allogeneic marrow. N Engl J Med 1969;281:691–7.
74. Vossen JM, de Koning J, van Bekkum DW, et al. Successful treatment of an infant with severe combined immunodeficiency by transplantation of bone marrow cells from an uncle. Clin Exp Immunol 1973;13:9–20.
75. O'Reilly RJ, Dupont B, Pahwa S, et al. Reconstitution in severe combined immunodeficiency by transplantation of marrow from an unrelated donor. N Engl J Med 1977;297:1311–8.
76. Reisner Y, Kirkpatrick D, Dupont B, et al. Transplantation for acute leukaemia with HLA-A and B nonidentical parental marrow cells fractionated with soybean agglutinin and sheep red blood cells. Lancet 1981;318:327–31.
77. Reisner Y, Kapoor N, Kirkpatrick D, et al. Transplantation for severe combined immunodeficiency with HLA-A, B, D, DR incompatible parental marrow cells fractionated by soybean agglutinin and sheep red blood cells. Blood 1983;61:341–8.
78. Haddad E, Allakhverdi Z, Griffith LM, et al. Survey on retransplantation criteria for patients with severe combined immunodeficiency. J Allergy Clin Immunol 2014;133:597–9.
79. Haddad E, Leroy S, Buckley RH. B-cell reconstitution for SCID: Should a conditioning regimen be used in SCID treatment? J Allergy Clin Immunol 2013;131(4):994–1000.
80. Buckley RH, Win CM, Moser BK, et al. Post-Transplantation B Cell Function in Different Molecular Types of SCID. J Clin Immunol 2013;33(1):96–110.

81. Grunebaum E, Roifman CM. Bone marrow transplantation using HLA-matched unrelated donors for patients suffering from severe combined immunodeficiency. Hematol Oncol Clin North Am 2011;25:63–73.

82. Dvorak CC, Hassan A, Slatter MA, et al. Comparison of outcomes of hematopoietic stem cell transplantation without chemotherapy conditioning by using matched sibling and unrelated donors for treatment of severe combined immunodeficiency. J Allergy Clin Immunol 2014;134:935–43.e15.

83. Hassan A, Lee P, Maggina P, et al. Host natural killer immunity is a key indicator of permissiveness for donor cell engraftment in patients with severe combined immunodeficiency. J Allergy Clin Immunol 2014;133:1660–6.

84. Keller MD, Chen DF, Condron SA, et al. The effect of natural killer cell killer Ig-like receptor alloreactivity on the outcome of bone marrow stem cell transplantation for severe combined immunodeficiency (SCID). J Clin Immunol 2007;27:109–16.

85. Kamili QUA, Seeborg FO, Saxena K, et al. Severe cutaneous human papillomavirus infection associated with natural killer cell deficiency following stem cell transplantation for severe combined immunodeficiency. J Allergy Clin Immunol 2014;134:1451–3.e1.

86. Laffort C, Deist FL, Favre M, et al. Severe cutaneous papillomavirus disease after haemopoietic stem-cell transplantation in patients with severe combined immune deficiency caused by common γc cytokine receptor subunit or JAK-3 deficiency. Lancet 2004;363:2051–4.

87. Koppelmans V, Breteler MMB, Boogerd W, et al. Neuropsychological performance in survivors of breast cancer more than 20 years after adjuvant chemotherapy. J Clin Oncol 2012;30(10):1080–6.

88. Titman P, Pink E, Skucek E, et al. Cognitive and behavioral abnormalities in children after hematopoietic stem cell transplantation for severe congenital immunodeficiencies. Blood 2008;112:3907–13.

89. Rogers MH, Lwin R, Fairbanks L, et al. Cognitive and behavioral abnormalities in adenosine deaminase deficient severe combined immunodeficiency. J Pediatr 2001;139:44–50.

90. Railey MD, Lokhnygina Y, Buckley RH. Long-term clinical outcome of patients with severe combined immunodeficiency who received related donor bone marrow transplants without pretransplant chemotherapy or post-transplant GVHD prophylaxis. J Pediatr 2009;155:834–40.e1.

91. Buckley R. Transplantation of hematopoietic stem cells in human severe combined immunodeficiency: long-term outcomes. Immunol Res 2011;49:25–43.

92. Myers LA, Patel DD, Puck JM, et al. Hematopoietic stem cell transplantation for severe combined immunodeficiency in the neonatal period leads to superior thymic output and improved survival. Blood 2002;99:872–8.

93. Onodera M, Ariga T, Kawamura N, et al. Successful peripheral T-lymphocyte–directed gene transfer for a patient with severe combined immune deficiency caused by adenosine deaminase deficiency. Blood 1998;91:30–6.

94. Kohn DB, Weinberg KI, Nolta JA, et al. Engraftment of gene-modified umbilical cord blood cells in neonates with adenosine deaminase deficiency. Nat Med 1995;1:1017–23.

95. Bordignon C, Notarangelo LD, Nobili N, et al. Gene therapy in peripheral blood lymphocytes and bone marrow for ADA negative immunodeficient patients. Science 1995;270:470.

96. Hoogerbrugge PM, van Beusechem VW, Fischer A, et al. Bone marrow gene transfer in three patients with adenosine deaminase deficiency. Gene Ther 1996;3:179–83.

97. Hacein-Bey-Abina S, Von Kalle C, Schmidt M, et al. LMO2-associated clonal T cell proliferation in two patients after gene therapy for SCID-X1. Science 2003; 302:415–9.

98. Hacein-Bey-Abina S, Garrigue A, Wang GP, et al. Insertional oncogenesis in 4 patients after retrovirus-mediated gene therapy of SCID-X1. J Clin Invest 2008;118:3132–42.

99. Howe SJ, Mansour MR, Schwarzwaelder K, et al. Insertional mutagenesis combined with acquired somatic mutations causes leukemogenesis following gene therapy of SCID-X1 patients. J Clin Invest 2008;118:3143–50.

100. Cappelli B, Aiuti A. Gene therapy for adenosine deaminase deficiency. Immunol Allergy Clin North Am 2010;30:249–60.

101. Gaspar HB, Cooray S, Gilmour KC, et al. Hematopoietic stem cell gene therapy for adenosine deaminase–deficient severe combined immunodeficiency leads to long-term immunological recovery and metabolic correction. Sci Transl Med 2011;3:97ra80.

102. Candotti F, Shaw KL, Muul L, et al. Gene therapy for adenosine deaminase-deficient severe combined immune deficiency: clinical comparison of retroviral vectors and treatment plans. Blood 2012;120(18):3635–46.

103. Thrasher AJ, Hacein-Bey-Abina S, Gaspar HB, et al. Failure of SCID-X1 gene therapy in older patients. Blood 2005;105:4255–7.

104. Hacein-Bey-Abina S, Pai S-Y, Gaspar HB, et al. A modified γ-retrovirus vector for X-linked severe combined immunodeficiency. N Engl J Med 2014;371:1407–17.

105. Naldini L, Blomer U, Gallay P, et al. In vivo gene delivery and stable transduction of nondividing cells by a lentiviral vector. Science 1996;272:263.

106. Zufferey R, Dull T, Mandel RJ, et al. Self-inactivating lentivirus vector for safe and efficient in vivo gene delivery. J Virol 1998;72:9873–80.

107. DiGeorge AM. Discussion of Cooper MD, Peterson RDA, Good RA. A new concept of cellular basis of immunity. J Pediatr 1965;67:907.

108. Conley ME, Beckwith JB, Mancer JFK, et al. The spectrum of the DiGeorge syndrome. J Pediatr 1979;94:883–90.

109. Barrett DJ, Ammann AJ, Wara DW, et al. Clinical and immunologic spectrum of the DiGeorge syndrome. J Clin Lab Immunol 1981;6:1–6.

110. Hong R. The DiGeorge anomaly. Immunodefic Rev 1991;3:1–14.

111. DiGeorge AM. Maldescent of the thymus. Pediatr Pathol 1994;14:178 [author reply: 9–80].

112. Rope AF, Cragun DL, Saal HM, et al. DiGeorge anomaly in the absence of chromosome 22q11.2 deletion. J Pediatr 2009;155:560–5.e1.

113. Markert M. Thymus transplantation. In: Sullivan K, Stiehm E, editors. Stiehm's immune deficiencies. 1st edition. Waltham (MA): Academic Press; 2014. p. 1059–67.

114. Markert M. Defects in thymic development: DiGeorge/CHARGE/chromosome 22q11.2 deletion. In: Sullivan K, Stiehm E, editors. Stiehm's immune deficiencies. 1st edition. Waltham (MA): Academic Press; 2014. p. 221–42.

115. Lingman Framme J, Borte S, von Döbeln U, et al. Retrospective analysis of TREC based newborn screening results and clinical phenotypes in infants with the 22q11 deletion syndrome. J Clin Immunol 2014;34:514–9.

116. Flanagan SP. 'Nude', a new hairless gene with pleiotropic effects in mouse. Genet Res 1966;8:295–309.

117. Pantelouris EM. Absence of thymus in a mouse mutant. Nature 1968;217:370–1.

118. Nehls M, Pfeifer D, Schorpp M, et al. New member of the winged-helix protein family disrupted in mouse and rat nude mutations. Nature 1994;372:103–7.

119. Frank J, Pignata C, Panteleyev AA, et al. Exposing the human nude phenotype. Nature 1999;398:473–4.

120. Pignata C, Fiore M, Guzzetta V, et al. Congenital alopecia and nail dystrophy associated with severe functional T-cell immunodeficiency in two sibs. Am J Med Genet 1996;65:167–70.

121. Markert ML, Hummell DS, Rosenblatt HM, et al. Complete DiGeorge syndrome: persistence of profound immunodeficiency. J Pediatr 1998;132:15–21.

122. Markert ML, Marques JG, Neven B, et al. First use of thymus transplantation therapy for FOXN1 deficiency (nude/SCID): a report of 2 cases. Blood 2011; 117:688–96.

123. Markert ML, Alexieff MJ, Li J, et al. Postnatal thymus transplantation with immunosuppression as treatment for DiGeorge syndrome. Blood 2004;104:2574–81.

124. Markert ML, Alexieff MJ, Li J, et al. Complete DiGeorge syndrome: development of rash, lymphadenopathy, and oligoclonal T cells in 5 cases. J Allergy Clin Immunol 2004;113:734–41.

125. Markert ML, Devlin BH, Alexieff MJ, et al. Review of 54 patients with complete DiGeorge anomaly enrolled in protocols for thymus transplantation: outcome of 44 consecutive transplants. Blood 2007;109:4539–47.

126. Chinn IK, Milner JD, Scheinberg P, et al. Thymus transplantation restores the repertoires of forkhead box protein 3 (FoxP3)+ and FoxP3−T cells in complete DiGeorge anomaly. Clin Exp Immunol 2013;173:140–9.

127. Markert ML, Devlin BH, Chinn IK, et al. Factors affecting success of thymus transplantation for complete DiGeorge anomaly. Am J Transplant 2008;8: 1729–36.

128. Chinn IK, Devlin BH, Li Y-J, et al. Long-term tolerance to allogeneic thymus transplants in complete DiGeorge anomaly. Clin Immunol 2008; 126:277–81.

129. Chinn IK, Olson JA, Skinner MA, et al. Mechanisms of tolerance to parental parathyroid tissue when combined with human allogeneic thymus transplantation. J Allergy Clin Immunol 2010;126:814–20.

130. Zheng P, Norosk LM, Hanson IC, et al. Molecular mechanisms of functional natural killer deficiency in patients with partial DiGeorge syndrome. J Allergy Clin Immunol 2015;135(5):1293–302.

131. Daguindau N, Decot V, Nzietchueng R, et al. Immune constitution monitoring after PBMC transplantation in complete DiGeorge syndrome: an eight-year follow-up. Clin Immunol 2008;128:164–71.

132. Land MH, Garcia-Lloret MI, Borzy MS, et al. Long-term results of bone marrow transplantation in complete DiGeorge syndrome. J Allergy Clin Immunol 2007; 120:908–15.

133. Bensoussan D, Le Deist F, Latger-Cannard V, et al. T-cell immune constitution after peripheral blood mononuclear cell transplantation in complete DiGeorge syndrome. Br J Haematol 2002;117:899–906.

134. Inoue H, Takada H, Kusuda T, et al. Successful cord blood transplantation for a CHARGE syndrome with CHD7 mutation showing DiGeorge sequence including hypoparathyroidism. Eur J Pediatr 2010;169:839–44.

135. Bowers DC, Lederman HM, Sicherer SH, et al. Immune constitution of complete DiGeorge anomaly by transplantation of unmobilised blood mononuclear cells. Lancet 1998;352:1983–4.

136. Janda A, Sedlacek P, Hönig M, et al. Multicenter survey on the outcome of transplantation of hematopoietic cells in patients with the complete form of DiGeorge anomaly. Blood 2010;116:2229–36.

137. Mazzolari E, Forino C, Guerci S, et al. Long-term immune reconstitution and clinical outcome after stem cell transplantation for severe T-cell immunodeficiency. J Allergy Clin Immunol 2007;120:892–9.

138. Markert ML. Treatment of infants with complete DiGeorge anomaly. J Allergy Clin Immunol 2008;121:1063.

139. Chan K, Puck JM. Development of population-based newborn screening for severe combined immunodeficiency. J Allergy Clin Immunol 2005;115:391–8.

140. Kubiak C, Jyonouchi S, Kuo C, et al. Fiscal implications of newborn screening in the diagnosis of severe combined immunodeficiency. J Allergy Clin Immunol 2014;2:697–702.

141. Modell V, Knaus M, Modell F. An analysis and decision tool to measure cost benefit of newborn screening for severe combined immunodeficiency (SCID) and related T-cell lymphopenia. Immunol Res 2014;60:145–52.

142. Routes JM, Grossman WJ, Verbsky J, et al. Statewide newborn screening for severe T-cell lymphopenia. JAMA 2009;302:2465–70.

143. Kwan A, Abraham RS, Currier R, et al. Newborn screening for severe combined immunodeficiency in 11 screening programs in the United States. JAMA 2014; 312:729–38.

144. Heimall J, Keller M, Saltzman R, et al. Diagnosis of 22q11.2 deletion syndrome and artemis deficiency in two children with T-B-NK+ immunodeficiency. J Clin Immunol 2012;32:1141–4.

145. Borte S, Wang N, Óskarsdóttir S, et al. Newborn screening for primary immunodeficiencies: beyond SCID and XLA. Ann N Y Acad Sci 2011;1246:118–30.

146. Turul T, Tezcan I, Artac H, et al. Clinical heterogeneity can hamper the diagnosis of patients with ZAP70 deficiency. Eur J Pediatr 2009;168:87–93.

147. Gadola SD, Moins-Teisserenc HT, Trowsdale J, et al. TAP deficiency syndrome. Clin Exp Immunol 2000;121:173–8.

148. Furukawa H, Murata S, Yabe T, et al. Splice acceptor site mutation of the transporter associated with antigen processing-1 gene in human bare lymphocyte syndrome. J Clin Invest 1999;103:755–8.

149. Klein C, Lisowska-Grospierre B, LeDeist F, et al. Major histocompatibility complex class II deficiency: clinical manifestations, immunologic features, and outcome. J Pediatr 1993;123:921–8.

150. Steimle V, Otten LA, Zufferey M, et al. Complementation cloning of an MHC class II transactivator mutated in hereditary MHC class II deficiency (or bare lymphocyte syndrome). Cell 1993;75:135–46.

151. Nagarajan UM, Louis-Plence P, DeSandro A, et al. RFX-B is the gene responsible for the most common cause of the bare lymphocyte syndrome, an MHC class II immunodeficiency. Immunity 1999;10:153–62.

152. Ouederni M, Vincent QB, Frange P, et al. Major histocompatibility complex class II expression deficiency caused by a RFXANK founder mutation: a survey of 35 patients. Blood 2011;118:5108–18.

153. Masternak K, Barras E, Zufferey M, et al. A gene encoding a novel RFX-associated transactivator is mutated in the majority of MHC class II deficiency patients. Nat Genet 1998;20:273–7.

154. Steimle V, Durand B, Barras E, et al. A novel DNA-binding regulatory factor is mutated in primary MHC class II deficiency (bare lymphocyte syndrome). Genes Development 1995;9:1021–32.

155. Durand B, Sperisen P, Emery P, et al. RFXAP, a novel subunit of the RFX DNA binding complex is mutated in MHC class II deficiency. EMBO J 1997;16:1045–55.

156. Engelhardt KR, McGhee S, Winkler S, et al. Large deletions and point mutations involving the dedicator of cytokinesis 8 (DOCK8) in the autosomal-recessive form of hyper-IgE syndrome. J Allergy Clin Immunol 2009;124:1289–302.e4.
157. Zhang Q, Davis JC, Lamborn IT, et al. Combined immunodeficiency associated with DOCK8 mutations. New Engl J Med 2009;361:2046–55.
158. Hauck F, Randriamampita C, Martin E, et al. Primary T-cell immunodeficiency with immunodysregulation caused by autosomal recessive LCK deficiency. J Allergy Clin Immunol 2012;130:1144–52.e11.
159. Goldman FD, Ballas ZK, Schutte BC, et al. Defective expression of p56lck in an infant with severe combined immunodeficiency. J Clin Invest 1998; 102:421–9.
160. Feske S, Picard C, Fischer A. Immunodeficiency due to mutations in ORAI1 and STIM1. Clin Immunol 2010;135:169–82.
161. Feske S, Gwack Y, Prakriya M, et al. A mutation in Orai1 causes immune deficiency by abrogating CRAC channel function. Nature 2006;441:179–85.
162. Picard C, McCarl C-A, Papolos A, et al. STIM1 mutation associated with a syndrome of immunodeficiency and autoimmunity. New Engl J Med 2009;360: 1971–80.
163. Keller MD, Ganesh J, Heltzer M, et al. Severe combined immunodeficiency resulting from mutations in MTHFD1. Pediatrics 2013;131:e629–34.
164. Borzutzky A, Crompton B, Bergmann AK, et al. Reversible severe combined immunodeficiency phenotype secondary to a mutation of the proton-coupled folate transporter. Clin Immunol 2009;133:287–94.

Hematopoietic Stem Cell Transplant for Immune Deficiency and Immune Dysregulation Disorders

David Hagin, MD, PhD[a,b,c], Lauri Burroughs, MD[a,b,d],
Troy R. Torgerson, MD, PhD[a,b,c],*

KEYWORDS

• PIDD • HSCT • BMT • Conditioning • GVHD • GVT • Rejection

KEY POINTS

- Hematopoietic stem cell transplant (HSCT) is a curative therapy for many immunodeficiency/immune dysregulation disorders.
- Three major factors need to be addressed when considering HSCT: donor stem cell source, conditioning regimen, and graft-versus-host disease (GVHD) prophylaxis.
- In general, the risks of graft rejection and GVHD are proportional to the degree of HLA mismatch between the donor and the recipient.
- In general, the risk of toxicity and death from infection is proportional to the intensity of the pretransplant conditioning regimen.
- The appropriate HSCT regimen varies depending on the immunodeficiency being treated and must balance donor stem cell availability and intensity of the conditioning regimen with risks including death from infection or toxicity, possibility of graft rejection, and the chance of GVHD.

INTRODUCTION

Primary immunodeficiency disorders (PIDDs) are a group of heterogeneous diseases, many of which are caused by monogenic defects, resulting in susceptibility to life-threatening infections, uncontrolled inflammation, or autoimmunity. As most immune

[a] Seattle Children's Hospital, 4800 Sand Point Way NE, Seattle, WA 98105, USA; [b] University of Washington School of Medicine, 1959 NE Pacific St, Seattle, WA 98195, USA; [c] Seattle Children's Research Institute, 1900 9th Avenue, JMB-7, Seattle, WA 98101-1304, USA; [d] Fred Hutchinson Cancer Research Center, 1100 Fairview Avenue North, Suite D3-100, Seattle, WA 98109, USA
* Corresponding author. Seattle Children's Research Institute, 1900 9th Avenue, JMB-7, Seattle, WA 98101-1304.
E-mail address: troy.torgerson@seattlechildrens.org

Immunol Allergy Clin N Am 35 (2015) 695–711
http://dx.doi.org/10.1016/j.iac.2015.07.010
immunology.theclinics.com

cells are derived from hematopoietic stem cells, HSCTs have long been considered a possible curative treatment of PIDDs.

In the late 1960s the fields of clinical immunology and bone marrow transplant became inseparably connected with the publication of the first successful bone marrow transplants for PIDD. Work had been underway for some time to develop a successful approach to perform HSCTs, but of the first 200 patients treated between 1957 and 1967, including 12 patients with immunodeficiency disorders, none survived the procedure.[1] The concept of HLA matching was in its infancy, so patients succumbed most commonly to graft rejection and GVHD. In 1968, 2 patients with PIDD underwent successful transplant: one for severe combined immunodeficiency (SCID)[2] and the other for Wiskott-Aldrich syndrome (WAS).[3] These cases represented the first successful HSCT procedures, changing forever how PIDD would be treated and ushering in the era of curative therapies for these disorders.

Over time, approaches to improve donor cell engraftment and decrease transplant-related mortality related to infections, organ dysfunction, and GVHD have led to progressively better HSCT outcomes; this has been driven by advances in 3 major technical aspects of HSCT, each of which are addressed in this article:

1. Selection of a suitable donor to provide stem cells capable of successfully engrafting, curing the underlying disease, and avoiding extensive reaction against the host (GVHD).
2. Selection of a conditioning regimen capable of opening sufficient space in the bone marrow to allow engraftment without creating severe life-threatening side effects.
3. Selection of a posttransplant immunosuppressive regimen capable of a preventing GVHD while allowing engraftment and expansion of donor cells.

Although there have been significant advances in the field, ongoing work continues to focus on improving and refining each of these 3 key aspects of the transplant approach.

IMPORTANT POINTS TO CONSIDER WHEN CONTEMPLATING HEMATOPOIETIC STEM CELL TRANSPLANT FOR PRIMARY IMMUNODEFICIENCY DISORDER

Unlike malignant diseases, in which transplant is a life-saving procedure applied primarily to allow the use of otherwise lethal doses of chemotherapy or radiation and to realize potential benefit from a graft-versus-tumor (GVT) effect, neither of these is important for patients with PIDD. Other key factors play a more significant role when considering HSCT for nonmalignant diseases such as PIDD.

In many patients with PIDD, an underlying molecular defect can be determined thus allowing a definitive diagnosis and providing some information regarding disease prognosis and potential utility of HSCT (**Table 1**). In these patients, it is relatively straightforward to proceed to transplant based on knowledge about the underlying disease. Problems arise, however, in patients who have a severe PIDD but lack a molecular diagnosis. Often in these cases, HSCT is delayed until the patient clearly demonstrates susceptibility to severe recurrent infections or autoimmunity, which can delay the decision to proceed to transplant for months to years. In these patients, the most important consideration before transplant is whether replacing the hematopoietic stem cells will be sufficient to cure or substantially improve the disorder. For example, in lymphocyte defects such as SCID, abnormalities are isolated almost exclusively to hematopoietic cells and HSCT can cure all aspects of the disease. There are, however, disorders that have a mixture of hematopoietic and nonhematopoietic defects such as autosomal dominant hyper-IgE syndrome (AD-HIES) caused by

Table 1 Immunodeficiency disorders and HSCT	
	References
HSCT Is Efficacious and Recommended	
CGD	4,5
DOCK8 deficiency	16
GATA2 deficiency	25,26
Griscelli syndrome, type II (RAB27A deficiency)	27,28
IPEX	29,30
LAD I, ITGB2 (CD18) deficiency	31,32
Perforin deficiency (PRF1 deficiency)	33,34
SCID	17,18
SCN	35,36
WAS	19,20
XHIM	37
XLP1 (SAP deficiency)	38
XLP2 (XIAP deficiency)	39,40
HSCT May Be Efficacious but Limited Evidence (<10 cases)	
Adenosine deaminase type II deficiency (DADA2)	41,42
AD-HIES	43,44
C1Q deficiency	45
CD25 deficiency	46
CTLA-4 haploinsufficiency	—
IL-10 deficiency	47,48
IL-10 receptor deficiency	47,48
LRBA deficiency	49
NBS	50
PGM3 deficiency	51
STAT1-GOF	52
STAT3-GOF	53
WHIM	54
HSCT Is Controversial	
CVID	55
DGS	56
IκBα deficiency (NFKBIA deficiency)	57,58
NEMO deficiency (IKBKG deficiency)	57,59
XLA	60
XLT, unless matched sibling available	61,62

Abbreviations: AD-HIES, autosomal dominant hyper-IgE syndrome; CGD, chronic granulomatous disease; CTLA-4, cytotoxic T-lymphocyte-associated protein 4; CVID, common variable immunodeficiency; DGS, DiGeorge syndrome; DOCK8, dedicator of cytokinesis 8; GOF, gain of function; IL, interleukin; IPEX, immune dysregulation, polyendocrinopathy, enteropathy, X-linked; LAD I, leukocyte adhesion deficiency, type I; LRBA, lipopolysaccharide responsive and beige-like anchor protein; NBS, Nijmegen breakage syndrome; PGM3, phosphoglucomutase 3; SCN, severe congenital neutropenia; STAT, signal transducer and activator of transcription; WHIM, warts, hypogammaglobulinemia, infections, myelokathexis; XHIM, X-linked hyper-IgM syndrome; XLA, X-linked agammaglobulinemia; XLP1, X-linked lyphoproliferative disease type I; XLP2, X-linked lyphoproliferative disease type II; XLT, X-linked thrombocytopenia.

Data from Refs.[4,5,16–20,25–62]

loss-of-function mutations in signal transducer and activator of transcription 3. In AD-HIES, HSCT can cure the defects in lymphocytes and myeloid cells but will likely not affect connective tissue abnormalities or vascular aneurysms, which are also characteristics of the disease. Similarly, there are immunodeficiencies such as DiGeorge syndrome in which the primary defect is in nonhematopoietic cells (thymus) and the role for HSCT remains controversial (see **Table 1**). In each case, the donor stem cell source, conditioning regimen, and GVHD prophylaxis approach need to be carefully considered to optimize the chances for a successful HSCT.

STEM CELL DONOR SELECTION

Proper donor selection is a key factor in preventing posttransplant GVHD and graft rejection. In HSCT for malignant diseases, some degree of donor-recipient mismatch may be acceptable because of the urgency and severity of the underlying disease; this may even have some advantage related to a GVT effect but is not the case for PIDDs. In patients with SCID HSCT is considered an urgent life-saving procedure, although there is typically at least some flexibility related to timing of transplant. In other PIDDs, wherein the underlying defect does not result in an imminent risk, HSCT can be delayed until a proper donor is found because the risk of GVHD can outweigh the benefit of HSCT.

Donor Types

There are 4 major donor types that are typically considered as a stem cell source for HSCT. Each has been used to treat patients with PIDDs and each has advantages and disadvantages that need to be considered in planning HSCT for a particular patient (**Table 2**).

Matched related donor
Matched related donor (MRD) is broadly considered to be the most desirable donor source. The most common MRD type is a fully matched sibling donor. In addition to

Table 2		
Advantages and disadvantages by stem cell donor source		
Regimen	**Advantages**	**Disadvantages**
MRD	• Donor is typically a sibling so is readily accessible. • Lowest risk for GVHD and graft failure	• Only ~30% chance for a recipient to have an MRD available
MUD	• Large database. • Outcomes nearly as good as MRD donors for many diseases	• Takes time to find a match (6–8 wk), so may delay an urgent transplant
CBD (cord)	• Cord blood units readily available in bank so can be obtained quickly • Generally more forgiving of HLA mismatches	• Requires MAC or near-MAC • Contains mostly naive cells so little preexisting viral immunity • Limited number of stem cells
MMRD (haplo)	• Readily available donor source for urgent transplant, parents at bedside	• Typically requires graft manipulation to deplete reactive T cells, etc. • Highest risk of graft rejection and GVHD

Abbreviations: CBD, cord blood donor; MAC, myeloablative conditioning; MMRD, mismatched related donor; MRD, matched related donor; MUD, matched unrelated donor.

matching at the major HLA alleles, MRDs have the advantage of a higher degree of matching at minor alleles. Therefore in most circumstances, matched sibling donors are assumed to have the lowest risk of all donor types for graft rejection and for GVHD. The circumstance in which a matched sibling donor is available to treat a patient with SCID is virtually the only situation in which HSCT is performed using an unmanipulated donor graft with no pretransplant conditioning. MRDs are particularly valuable for patients who have mixed racial or ethnic backgrounds and for those from ethnic groups that are not well represented in the unrelated bone marrow or cord blood donor (CBD) pool, because finding a suitable, fully matched donor is challenging and a matched sibling donor can be the only available donor option.

One consideration unique to the use of MRD in PIDD is donor disease status. Before using siblings as donors, it is important to assure that they do not harbor the same disease as the recipient. This process is straightforward if the causative genetic defect is known but much more complicated in the absence of an established underlying diagnosis. In addition, a significant debate remains regarding whether matched sibling donors who are carriers of a disease (eg, X-linked chronic granulomatous disease [CGD] carriers) should be considered as donors for affected siblings or not. This decision may vary depending on the underlying disease and the availability of alternative donors.

The most significant challenge related to the use of matched sibling donors is the lack of a sibling donor in most cases. Owing to the manner in which the HLA alleles are inherited, each sibling has a 25% chance of being matched to the recipient. For this reason, some families who have children with PIDD who need transplant may delay the transplant while they have additional children or may take advantage of pre-implantation genetic diagnosis and in vitro fertilization to select for a child that does not have the disease and is HLA matched to the recipient.

Matched unrelated donor
There are several hematopoietic stem cell registries that collect and catalog potential HSCT donors for transplant. The largest of these is the National Marrow Donor Program (NMDP) in the United States. The NMDP database in collaboration with other international registries provides access to over 24.5 million bone marrow donors and 622,000 cord blood units (http://bethematch.org). Despite this large number, there continue to be a significant percentage of patients who do not have access to a matched donor. This fact is particularly true for patients of racially mixed backgrounds or ethnic minorities for whom there are fewer donors with similar backgrounds in the database.

In recently published transplant studies for SCID, WAS, CGD, and other PIDDs, survival using matched unrelated donors (MUD) approaches the results obtained using matched sibling donors. MUD is therefore considered by many to be the next best alternative to an MRD.[4,5] Despite this, one significant disadvantage of MUD is the duration of the search procedure. In preparation for transplant, the databases are searched and the NMDP then coordinates the collection of blood from potential donors to perform high-resolution HLA typing studies. Sometimes in the process, donors presumed to be a match based on the preliminary typing result in the database are found to be incompatible on further testing. Once a specific donor is identified and confirmed to be compatible, the NMDP coordinates the collection of donor stem cells and the transplant proceeds. This process can take several weeks, a major disadvantage if a patient is acutely ill and requires an urgent transplant (ie, a patient with SCID with infections).

Cord blood donor

As noted above, the NMDP maintains a large database of cord blood units available for HSCT. The major advantage of cord blood is that it is available off the shelf, so it can be obtained almost immediately. As a general rule, cord blood also tends to be more forgiving of HLA mismatches than bone marrow or peripheral blood from a more mature donor. The major disadvantages of cord blood are 3-fold. First, several studies have made it clear that engraftment of cord blood stem cells is most successful following myeloablative conditioning (MAC) and that the success rate of engraftment decreases with the reduction in the intensity of the conditioning regimen.[6] In the setting of a patient with PIDD who may have preexisting infections or organ dysfunction, MAC can substantially increase the risk of morbidity and mortality. Second, cord blood cells are largely naive, so little to no antiviral immunity is transferred to the donor cells. Also, immune reconstitution in recipients of CBD was shown to be slower than that in recipients of unmanipulated bone marrow.[7] As a result, cord blood may not be a good option for patients with active viral infections or in patients who are predicted to have poor thymic function based on their underlying molecular defect. Third, because there is a finite volume of blood in a cord blood sample, the number of $CD34^+$ stem cells available to transplant is limited. As the time to engraftment and the speed of cellular recovery posttransplant correlates with the number of transplanted stem cells, recent recommendations have suggested using a minimum total nucleated cell dose of 2×10^7 cells/kg or 2×10^5 $CD34^+$ stem cells/kg,[8] but the acceptable minimum cell dose depends on the degree of mismatching. This means that an average single cord blood unit is often sufficient only for patients weighing up to approximately 30 kg. As a result, there have been an increasing number of transplants in larger patients using 2 unrelated cord blood units. In these cases, one of the cord blood units typically wins out and predominates the engraftment.

Mismatched related donor

The most commonly used mismatched related donor (MMRD) is a haploidentical parent. In some patients who have rare HLA haplotypes, a haploidentical transplant may be the best option if there are no acceptable MUD donors available. The risk for graft rejection and GVHD is high in a haploidentical transplant (**Fig. 1**) due largely to the presence of mismatched T cells. To decrease this risk, haploidentical samples need to be depleted of donor T cells either by depleting the T cells or by enriching the $CD34^+$ stem cells and leaving the T cells behind (see section on Graft Manipulation). Recent haploidentical transplant approaches have successfully used in vivo T-cell depletion by administering cyclophosphamide at days 3 and 4 posttransplant to deplete strongly alloreactive cells that have been activated at the time of transplant and are in the midst of strong proliferation.[9] The major advantage of using a haploidentical stem cell source is that typically one of the parents or a sibling is readily available to use as a donor.

Bone Marrow Versus Mobilized Peripheral Blood Stem Cells

For MRDs, MUDs, and MMRDs, there is an option to use either bone marrow or peripheral blood as a stem cell source. In order to use peripheral blood, the stem cells

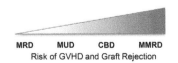

Fig. 1. Risk of GVHD and graft rejection increases according to donor stem cell source.

need to be mobilized from the bone marrow into the circulation. Traditionally, this is done by pretreating the donor for 4 to 6 days with granulocyte colony-stimulating factor before harvesting peripheral blood for transplant. There are, however, newer agents such as the CXCR4 antagonist plerixafor (AMD3100) that have shown promise in facilitating a more rapid mobilization of stem cells, but these are not yet routinely used in most centers.[10]

Both bone marrow and mobilized peripheral blood stem cells (PBSCs) have been used successfully for HSCT in PIDD, but each has its own advantages and disadvantages that should be considered. Peripheral blood has the potential to deliver a larger cell dose per kilogram than may be achievable with bone marrow cells and as a result may promote engraftment and facilitate immune reconstitution in patients who receive minimal-intensity conditioning regimens. The downside of PBSC grafts is that within the large number of cells that can be delivered, there are also a larger number of mature alloreactive effector cells, and therefore, higher rates of GVHD are common.[11]

Stem Cell Graft Manipulation

As noted above, the use of an MMRD requires manipulation of the donor stem cells before or after transplant to decrease the risk of graft rejection and GVHD. Traditionally, this was accomplished by agglutination of T cells on soybean lectin and E-rosetting on sheep red blood cells.[12,13] Technological advances using a variety of approaches including antibody-coated magnetic beads have allowed this to be done in a much more specific and selective manner. At present, the most widely used approaches involve selected isolation of CD34$^+$ stem cells from the bone marrow or peripheral blood using magnetic particles coated with antibodies against CD34. Frequently, this approach yields CD34$^+$ stem cells of such high purity that small numbers of donor T cells need to be added back to the purified stem cells to promote engraftment in the recipient. These approaches continue to be refined, and recently, excellent success has been achieved in nonmalignant transplants using haploidentical stem cells depleted only of αβ T cells and CD19$^+$ B cells.[14] This approach leaves γδ T cells and natural killer (NK) cells in the donor graft, allowing control of intercurrent infections but minimizing the risk for GVHD.[15,16]

CONDITIONING REGIMEN

Variability in the underlying molecular cause of disease in various PIDDs dictates that a disease-specific approach to conditioning should be taken. In some PIDDs such as DNA repair disorders, the molecular defect that causes immunodeficiency also results in radiation sensitivity, so radiation therapy should be avoided or used with caution. In severe defects such as SCID, there is lower risk for graft rejection because of the profound underlying immune dysfunction, while in other less-severe defects (eg, WAS), a more intense conditioning regimen is required to allow engraftment and prevent rejection or to achieve high-level donor chimerism and prevent theoretic disease relapse caused by residual host cells (eg, hemophagocytic lymphohistiocytosis syndromes). It has become apparent therefore that not every PIDD responds equivalently to a particular transplant regimen and that a disease-specific approach offers the best chance for a successful HSCT outcome.

Myeloablative Conditioning Agents Versus Immunosuppressive Conditioning Agents

Virtually all bone marrow transplant conditioning regimens combine drugs or treatments that have myeloablative activity to open space in the bone marrow and allow donor cell engraftment, together with drugs that have immunosuppressive activity to prevent graft rejection by residual host cells and GVHD by transplanted and emerging donor cells. Commonly used myeloablative drugs include the alkylating agents busulfan and treosulfan. Commonly used immunosuppressive drugs include cyclophosphamide, fludarabine, and antibody-mediated cell-depleting agents including antithymocyte globulin (ATG) and alemtuzumab. Examples of drugs and treatments that have both activities include melphalan, thiotepa, and total body irradiation (TBI, depending on the dose used).

The intensity of the conditioning protocol should be disease oriented. In some PIDDs such as DNA repair disorders, the molecular defect that causes immunodeficiency also results in radiation sensitivity, and therefore radiation therapy should be avoided or used with caution in these patients. In more severe defects, one could expect a reduced risk for graft rejection by abnormal immune cells (SCID), whereas in others, a more intense protocol is required to allow engraftment and prevent rejection (eg, WAS) or to achieve high percent of donor chimerism and prevent theoretic disease relapse caused by residual host cells (eg, hemophagocytic lymphohistiocytosis syndrome). Therefore, a disease-specific approach should be adopted.

No Conditioning

Transplant regimens using no conditioning are reserved almost exclusively for patients with SCID in which the barriers to engraftment are minimal and the risk for graft rejection is low. As no conditioning is used, there is no risk for regimen-related toxicity (**Fig. 2**). The classic nonconditioned regimen for SCID involves use of a T-cell-depleted haploidentical graft. The disadvantage of this regimen is that patients often do not achieve complete, multilineage engraftment, particularly of B cells, and require ongoing IgG supplementation. In addition, over time, many patients show evidence for abnormal T-cell engraftment, reflected by lower numbers of naive CD4$^+$ T cells and chronic human papillomavirus infection.[17] One recent study further dissected different SCID syndromes based on their permissiveness for donor cell engraftment and suggested that nonconditioned regimens should be limited to NK-negative SCID.[18]

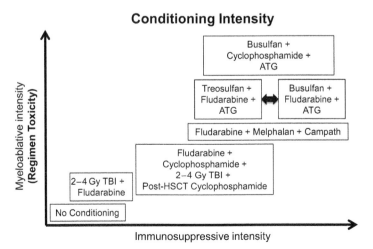

Fig. 2. Relative myeloablative and immunosuppressive capacity of common HSCT conditioning regimens. TBI - total body irradiation; ATG - anti-thymocyte globulin.

Minimal Intensity Conditioning

Minimal intensity conditioning (MIC) regimens often use only immunosuppressive agents (fludarabine, low-dose TBI, etc.) to minimize the recipient immune response to the transplanted graft. Because the agents and doses used have a relatively low risk of side effects, regimen-related toxicity in MIC regimens is quite low (see **Fig. 2**). This conditioning approach is used almost exclusively with matched sibling (MRD) or well-matched unrelated (MUD) donors as well as with select haploidentical transplant regimens. Often, a high dose of donor cell is used in an effort to drive-in a donor graft, as described above. This process may require the use of PBSC as opposed to bone marrow as a stem cell source, which is accompanied by an increased risk for GVHD.

Reduced Intensity Conditioning

There is a broad spectrum of intensity among conditioning regimens that are considered to be reduced intensity depending on the combination and doses of the agents used (see **Fig. 2**). The risk of regimen-related toxicity is generally proportionate to the intensity of the regimen. As many PIDDs do not require full donor chimerism to achieve functional reconstitution of immunity (eg, SCID; CGD; immune dysregulation, polyendocrinopathy, enteropathy, X-linked; X-linked hyper-IgM syndrome) there has been a move to use reduced intensity conditioning (RIC) regimens for many of these disorders. RIC has been used successfully with all donor stem cell sources, although cord blood typically requires a more aggressive RIC regimen to achieve stable engraftment. This approach provides an option for patients with PIDD who may have severe infections before transplant or may have preexisting risk factors such as lung, liver, or renal disease that would preclude them from undergoing transplant with a more aggressive conditioning regimen.

Myeloablative Conditioning

MAC is the most intense form of conditioning for HSCT and as a consequence bears the greatest risk for regimen-related toxicity (see **Fig. 2**). The classic MAC regimen combines myeloablative doses of busulfan with cyclophosphamide and ATG. Commonly referred to as Bu-Cy-ATG, this regimen has been used successfully to treat a broad range of immunodeficiency disorders. In many PIDDs, it has subsequently been recognized that a fully myeloablative regimen may not be required to achieve a stable donor graft. There are, however, immunodeficiencies such as WAS in which MAC regimens remain the preferred approach because of the need to achieve stable, high-level donor chimerism in both the lymphoid and myeloid compartments in order to cure the immunodeficiency, correct the platelet-based bleeding disorder, and prevent long-term autoimmunity.[19,20] In addition, MAC or near-MAC is generally required when using cord blood as a stem cell source.

GRAFT-VERSUS-HOST DISEASE AND PROPHYLAXIS

GVHD is one if the major complications that can occur after HSCT. In the setting of high-risk malignancy, survival benefits outweigh the risk of GVHD, which in fact may have a beneficial effect in helping to eradicate tumor cells through the immune response directed toward the host (GVT effect). In the setting of nonmalignant disorders such as PIDD, however, there is no benefit to GVHD, which in addition to affecting common target organs (liver, gastrointestinal tract, and skin) could delay desired post-transplant immune reconstitution and leave the patient susceptible to infection for a significant time after transplant.[21,22] As a rule, every effort is made to try and prevent GVHD in patients with PIDD. In addition to selecting the best matched donor or depleting donor T cells from the stem cell graft, GVHD prophylaxis takes 2 forms: (1) drugs administered during the conditioning process that have effects that extend beyond the transplant (ie, ATG or alemtuzumab administered near the transplant that continue to be present after transplant to ablate reactive lymphocytes in the graft) and (2) drugs administered after transplant, typically in tapering doses over the first several months, in an effort to prevent GVHD and graft rejection. These drugs include immunosuppressants such as cyclosporine, tacrolimus, sirolimus, methotrexate, and mycophenolate. Typically, the less intense the conditioning regimen, the more immunosuppression needs to be added as prophylaxis to prevent GVHD and graft rejection.

Although in most cases immunosuppressants are able to control GVHD, the nonselective nature of such treatments also results in some degree of graft suppression and delays immune reconstitution. Therefore, other methods are being developed to allow transfer of higher numbers of donor T cells while reducing the risk for GVHD without the use of long-term GVHD prophylaxis. Examples include the aforementioned $\alpha\beta$ T cells and CD19$^+$ B-cell depletion,[15] or the use of an engineered donor graft to include high numbers of donor regulatory T cells that effectively suppress GVHD.[23]

GRAFT FAILURE

The other major undesired outcome after transplant is graft failure in which donor stem cells either never engraft (primary graft failure) or engraft and then are lost over time (secondary graft failure). In most cases, this leads to repopulation with recipient cells, unless an MAC regimen was used in which case there is a risk of the patient becoming aplastic. Graft failure can result from a variety of factors including infections early after transplant (cytomegalovirus, human herpesvirus 6, parvovirus, etc.), drugs (ganciclovir, etc.), problems with the bone marrow stroma, or through immune-mediated processes related to HLA mismatches and alloantibodies. Graft failure caused by recipient cells attacking and destroying donor cells is called graft rejection.

Different methods can be used to prevent graft rejection, which in part parallel those used to prevent GVHD. These include selecting the best matched donor, escalating the donor stem cell dose, and using peritransplant immunosuppression. One additional intervention used in an effort to overcome decreasing donor engraftment (donor chimerism) in a posttransplant patient is the use of donor lymphocyte infusion in an attempt to tip the balance between donor cells and rejecting host cells. This intervention, however, is associated with a risk of promoting GVHD.

DONOR CHIMERISM

Donor chimerism refers to the percentage of cells in the recipient that are derived from the donor. The ideal outcome of every bone marrow transplant is to have full donor chimerism in every hematopoietic cell lineage at the conclusion of treatment. The reality, however, is that because of the use of RIC regimens and mismatched stem cell donors, many patients with immunodeficiencies have less than 100% donor chimerism in one or more cell lineages. The level of donor chimerism between different lineages can vary widely and in part depends on the underlying molecular defect. Often with more severe defects, healthy donor cells have a selective survival advantage, and higher levels of donor chimerism are expected mostly in the abnormal cell lineage. Although desired, full donor chimerism is not a requisite for successful PIDD transplant, because the level of donor chimerism in a key cell lineage required to cure a disorder also varies depending on the particular immunodeficiency being treated (such as in the case of CD40L deficiency mentioned below).

Assessment of Donor Chimerism

Donor chimerism can be evaluated in any subset of hematopoietic cells that can be isolated. Because of the cost and complexity involved in isolating various cell subsets, donor chimerism is often measured in whole blood (whole blood chimerism). In many clinical centers, donor chimerism is routinely assessed in both the myeloid and lymphoid compartments (myeloid vs lymphoid chimerism). In some centers, the lymphoid compartment is further subdivided and assessed individually in T cells, B cells, and NK cells. In PIDD, it is not uncommon to have split or mixed donor chimerism after HSCT as a result of engraftment of 1 cell compartment but not others, particularly in those patients treated with RIC regimens. One of the classic examples is X-linked SCID, a $T^{neg}B^+NK^{neg}$ form of SCID in which patients often have donor engraftment in the T-cell compartment, and to a lesser degree, the NK cell compartment but have no donor engraftment in the B-cell compartment. As a result, it is not uncommon for these patients to be cured of the usual clinical symptoms of SCID but still lack the ability to generate productive antibody responses to antigen challenge and thus require ongoing treatment with immunoglobulin replacement therapy. Because PIDD may be caused by defects in just one compartment of the immune system, it is particularly important in these diseases to be certain to assess donor chimerism and functional immune recovery in the key subset of cells that caused the disease. For example, in patients with CGD, myeloid donor chimerism and demonstration that neutrophils have a normal oxidative burst are the key determinants in assessing whether HSCT was successful.

Typically, there are 3 main methods of assessing donor chimerism:

1. Fluorescence in situ hybridization for sex chromosomes: this method depends on a sex mismatch between the donor and the recipient (ie, evaluating the percentage of female donor cells in a male recipient). This approach can be performed on a small number of cells, and it generates a highly accurate result because the cells are visually counted.
2. Variable number of tandem repeats and small tandem repeats testing are DNA-based approaches using polymerase chain reaction (PCR) to amplify segments of the genome known to be highly heterogeneous because of expansion of tandem repeats that differ from individual to individual. The amplified fragments are then resolved by electrophoresis. This approach is a standard one used by many chimerism laboratories to assess donor chimerism. One disadvantage is that the performing laboratory needs to have DNA stored from the donor to perform this analysis. As the method is performed by PCR, small numbers of cells can be analyzed. The electrophoresis step that follows, however, is not as sensitive and can make it difficult to accurately quantitate very low donor chimerism levels (<10%).
3. Evaluation of protein and/or functional recovery by flow cytometry: this approach is made possible by the fact that many patients with PIDD have genetic defects that lead to the absence or dysfunction of a particular protein in immune cells. For example, in patients who undergo HSCT for CGD, evaluation of the neutrophil oxidative burst by the dihydrorhodamine 123 assay can quickly determine the level of donor chimerism in neutrophils by comparing the percentage of cells that have a normal oxidative burst to the percentage that have a persistently abnormal oxidative burst. Similarly, in patients with WAS who have mutations that cause a lack of WASp protein expression, flow cytometry can be used to evaluate the percentage of cells that have normal WASp protein expression (donor cells) after HSCT. By including additional antibodies to cell surface markers such as CD4, CD8, CD19,

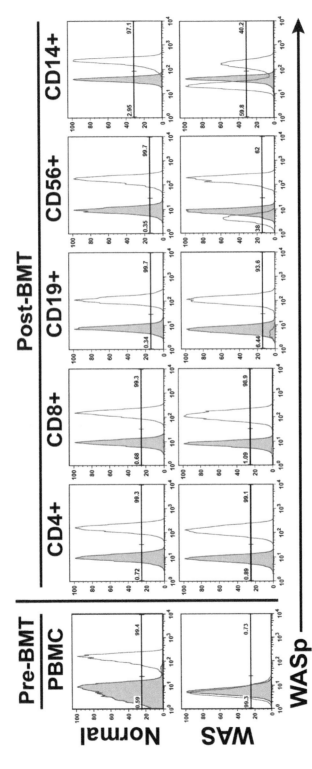

Fig. 3. Demonstration of performing functional donor chimerism in a male child with Wiskott-Aldrich syndrome. Cells were evaluated by flow cytometry after intracellular staining with a rabbit polyclonal antibody specific for the Wiskott-Aldrich Syndrome protein (WASp). Cells were co-stained for lineage-specific cell surface markers including CD4, CD8, CD19, CD56, and CD14. Note that after HSCT, the patient who had no WASp protein expression before transplant has full donor chimerism in T cells (CD4 and CD8) and B cells (CD19). NK cells (CD56) and Monocytes (CD14) show mixed donor chimerism. This result correlated with donor chimerism levels estimated by the variable number of tandem repeats/small tandem repeats method.

CD56, CD14, and CD42, WASp protein expression can be simultaneously evaluated in T cells, B cells, NK cells, monocyte/macrophages, and platelets, thus providing a rapid assessment of donor chimerism in all cell compartments without the need to sort or purify each cell subset **(Fig. 3)**.

SUMMARY

The fields of HSCT and primary immunodeficiency diseases have coevolved, and HSCT has become an indispensible tool as a curative therapy for PIDD. The breadth of immunodeficiency disorders treated by HSCT has continued to expand, and the approaches used to perform the transplants have continued to improve such that for some disorders, success rates are over 90%. However, there is an urgent need for the development of transplant approaches that are even safer as highlighted by the recent report of 2 patients with SCID successfully identified by SCID newborn screening who died as a consequence of complications related to the conditioning regimen used for HSCT.[24] This outcome is unacceptable because it negates the advantages in survival and outcome gained by the institution of SCID newborn screening in the first place. The development of improved approaches to conditioning will have the added benefit of paving the way for improved outcomes using the next generation of curative therapies including gene therapy and gene repair.

REFERENCES

1. Bortin MM. A compendium of reported human bone marrow transplants. Transplantation 1970;9(6):571–87.
2. Gatti R, Meuwissen H, Allen H, et al. Immunological reconstitution of sex-linked lymphopenic immunological deficiency. Lancet 1968;292(7583):1366–9.
3. Bach F, Albertini R, Joo P, et al. Bone-marrow transplantation in a patient with the Wiskott-Aldrich syndrome. Lancet 1968;292(7583):1364–6.
4. Martinez CA, Shah S, Shearer WT, et al. Excellent survival after sibling or unrelated donor stem cell transplantation for chronic granulomatous disease. J Allergy Clin Immunol 2012;129(1):176–83.
5. Güngör T, Teira P, Slatter M, et al. Reduced-intensity conditioning and HLA-matched haemopoietic stem-cell transplantation in patients with chronic granulomatous disease: a prospective multicentre study. Lancet 2014;383(9915):436–48.
6. Marsh RA, Rao MB, Gefen A, et al. Experience with alemtuzumab, fludarabine, and melphalan reduced-intensity conditioning hematopoietic cell transplantation in patients with nonmalignant diseases reveals good outcomes and that the risk of mixed chimerism depends on underlying disease, stem cell source, and alemtuzumab regimen. Biol Blood Marrow Transplant 2015;21(8):1460–70.
7. Komanduri KV, St John LS, de Lima M, et al. Delayed immune reconstitution after cord blood transplantation is characterized by impaired thymopoiesis and late memory T-cell skewing. Blood 2007;110(13):4543–51.
8. Welte K, Foeken L, Gluckman E, et al. International exchange of cord blood units: The registry aspects. Bone Marrow Transplant 2010;45(5):825–31.
9. Brunstein CG, Fuchs EJ, Carter SL, et al. Alternative donor transplantation after reduced intensity conditioning: results of parallel phase 2 trials using partially HLA-mismatched related bone marrow or unrelated double umbilical cord blood grafts. Blood 2011;118(2):282–8.
10. Devine SM, Vij R, Rettig M, et al. Rapid mobilization of functional donor hematopoietic cells without G-CSF using AMD3100, an antagonist of the CXCR4/SDF-1 interaction. Blood 2008;112(4):990–8.

11. Anasetti C, Logan BR, Lee SJ, et al. Peripheral-blood stem cells versus bone marrow from unrelated donors. N Engl J Med 2012;367(16):1487–96.
12. Reisner Y, Kapoor N, O'Reilly RJ, et al. Allogeneic bone marrow transplantation using stem cells fractionated by lectins: VI, in vitro analysis of human and monkey bone marrow cells fractionated by sheep red blood cells and soybean agglutinin. Lancet 1980;2(8208–8209):1320–4.
13. Reisner Y, Kapoor N, Kirkpatrick D, et al. Transplantation for severe combined immunodeficiency with HLA-A, B,D,DR incompatible parental marrow cells fractionated by soybean agglutinin and sheep red blood cells. Blood 1983;61(2): 341–8.
14. Schumm M, Lang P, Bethge W, et al. Depletion of T-cell receptor alpha/beta and CD19 positive cells from apheresis products with the CliniMACS device. Cytotherapy 2013;15(10):1253–8.
15. Lang P, Feuchtinger T, Teltschik H, et al. Improved immune recovery after transplantation of TCRαβ/CD19-depleted allografts from haploidentical donors in pediatric patients. Bone Marrow Transplant 2015;50:S6–10.
16. Ghosh S, Schuster FR, Adams O, et al. Haploidentical stem cell transplantation in DOCK8 deficiency - successful control of pre-existing severe viremia with a TCRass/CD19-depleted graft and antiviral treatment. Clin Immunol 2014; 152(1–2):111–4.
17. Neven B, Leroy S, Decaluwe H, et al. Long-term outcome after hematopoietic stem cell transplantation of a single-center cohort of 90 patients with severe combined immunodeficiency. Blood 2009;113(17):4114–24.
18. Hassan A, Lee P, Maggina P, et al. Host natural killer immunity is a key indicator of permissiveness for donor cell engraftment in patients with severe combined immunodeficiency. J Allergy Clin Immunol 2014;133(6):1660–6.
19. Ozsahin H, Cavazzana-Calvo M, Notarangelo LD, et al. Long-term outcome following hematopoietic stem-cell transplantation in Wiskott-Aldrich syndrome: collaborative study of the European Society for Immunodeficiencies and European Group for Blood and Marrow Transplantation. Blood 2008;111(1):439–45.
20. Moratto D, Giliani S, Bonfim C, et al. Long-term outcome and lineage-specific chimerism in 194 patients with Wiskott-Aldrich syndrome treated by hematopoietic cell transplantation in the period 1980-2009: an international collaborative study. Blood 2011;118(6):1675–84.
21. Clave E, Busson M, Douay C, et al. Acute graft-versus-host disease transiently impairs thymic output in young patients after allogeneic hematopoietic stem cell transplantation. Blood 2009;113(25):6477–84.
22. Cavazzana-Calvo M, Andre-Schmutz I, Dal Cortivo L, et al. Immune reconstitution after haematopoietic stem cell transplantation: obstacles and anticipated progress. Curr Opin Immunol 2009;21(5):544–8.
23. Di Ianni M, Falzetti F, Carotti A, et al. Tregs prevent GVHD and promote immune reconstitution in HLA-haploidentical transplantation. Blood 2011;117(14):3921–8.
24. Kwan A, Abraham RS, Currier R, et al. Newborn screening for severe combined immunodeficiency in 11 screening programs in the united states. JAMA 2014; 312(7):729–38.
25. Grossman J, Cuellar-Rodriguez J, Gea-Banacloche J, et al. Nonmyeloablative allogeneic hematopoietic stem cell transplantation for GATA2 deficiency. Biol Blood Marrow Transplant 2014;20(12):1940–8.
26. Cuellar-Rodriguez J, Gea-Banacloche J, Freeman AF, et al. Successful allogeneic hematopoietic stem cell transplantation for GATA2 deficiency. Blood 2011; 118(13):3715–20.

27. Rossi A, Borroni RG, Carrozzo AM, et al. Griscelli syndrome type 2: long-term follow-up after unrelated donor bone marrow transplantation. Dermatology 2009;218(4):376–9.
28. Schuster F, Stachel DK, Schmid I, et al. Griscelli syndrome: report of the first peripheral blood stem cell transplant and the role of mutations in the RAB27A gene as an indication for BMT. Bone Marrow Transplant 2001;28(4):409–12.
29. Burroughs LM, Torgerson TR, Storb R, et al. Stable hematopoietic cell engraftment after low-intensity nonmyeloablative conditioning in patients with immune dysregulation, polyendocrinopathy, enteropathy, X-linked syndrome. J Allergy Clin Immunol 2010;126(5):1000–5.
30. Rao A, Kamani N, Filipovich A, et al. Successful bone marrow transplantation for IPEX syndrome after reduced-intensity conditioning. Blood 2007;109(1):383–5.
31. Qasim W, Cavazzana-Calvo M, Davies EG, et al. Allogeneic hematopoietic stem-cell transplantation for leukocyte adhesion deficiency. Pediatrics 2009;123(3):836–40.
32. Thomas C, Le Deist F, Cavazzana-Calvo M, et al. Results of allogeneic bone marrow transplantation in patients with leukocyte adhesion deficiency. Blood 1995;86(4):1629–35.
33. Ouachée-Chardin M, Elie C, de Saint Basile G, et al. Hematopoietic stem cell transplantation in hemophagocytic lymphohistiocytosis: a single-center report of 48 patients. Pediatrics 2006;117(4):e743–50.
34. Filipovich AH. Life-threatening hemophagocytic syndromes: current outcomes with hematopoietic stem cell transplantation. Pediatr Transplant 2005;9(Suppl 7):87–91.
35. Connelly JA, Choi SW, Levine JE. Hematopoietic stem cell transplantation for severe congenital neutropenia. Curr Opin Hematol 2012;19(1):44–51.
36. Carlsson G, Winiarski J, Ljungman P, et al. Hematopoietic stem cell transplantation in severe congenital neutropenia. Pediatr Blood Cancer 2011;56(3):444–51.
37. Mitsui-Sekinaka K, Imai K, Sato H, et al. Clinical features and hematopoietic stem cell transplantation for CD40 ligand deficiency in Japan. J Allergy Clin Immunol 2015 [pii:S0091-6749(15)00269-9] [Epub ahead of print].
38. Booth C, Gilmour KC, Veys P, et al. X-linked lymphoproliferative disease due to SAP/SH2D1A deficiency: a multicenter study on the manifestations, management and outcome of the disease. Blood 2011;117(1):53–62.
39. Marsh RA, Kim MO, Liu C, et al. An intermediate alemtuzumab schedule reduces the incidence of mixed chimerism following reduced-intensity conditioning hematopoietic cell transplantation for hemophagocytic lymphohistiocytosis. Biol Blood Marrow Transplant 2013;19(11):1625–31.
40. Marsh RA, Rao K, Satwani P, et al. Allogeneic hematopoietic cell transplantation for XIAP deficiency: an international survey reveals poor outcomes. Blood 2013;121(6):877–83.
41. Van Eyck L Jr, Hershfield MS, Pombal D, et al. Hematopoietic stem cell transplantation rescues the immunologic phenotype and prevents vasculopathy in patients with adenosine deaminase 2 deficiency. J Allergy Clin Immunol 2015;135(1):283–7.e5.
42. van Montfrans J, Zavialov A, Zhou Q. Mutant ADA2 in vasculopathies. N Engl J Med 2014;371(5):478.
43. Patel NC, Gallagher JL, Torgerson TR, et al. Successful haploidentical donor hematopoietic stem cell transplant and restoration of STAT3 function in an adolescent with autosomal dominant hyper-IgE syndrome. J Clin Immunol 2015;35(5):479–85.

44. Goussetis E, Peristeri I, Kitra V, et al. Successful long-term immunologic reconstitution by allogeneic hematopoietic stem cell transplantation cures patients with autosomal dominant hyper-IgE syndrome. J Allergy Clin Immunol 2010;126(2): 392–4.
45. Arkwright PD, Riley P, Hughes SM, et al. Successful cure of C1q deficiency in human subjects treated with hematopoietic stem cell transplantation. J Allergy Clin Immunol 2014;133(1):265–7.
46. Roifman CM. Human IL-2 receptor alpha chain deficiency. Pediatr Res 2000; 48(1):6–11.
47. Engelhardt KR, Shah N, Faizura-Yeop I, et al. Clinical outcome in IL-10- and IL-10 receptor-deficient patients with or without hematopoietic stem cell transplantation. J Allergy Clin Immunol 2013;131(3):825–30.
48. Kotlarz D, Beier R, Murugan D, et al. Loss of interleukin-10 signaling and infantile inflammatory bowel disease: implications for diagnosis and therapy. Gastroenterology 2012;143(2):347–55.
49. Seidel MG, Hirschmugl T, Gamez-Diaz L, et al. Long-term remission after allogeneic hematopoietic stem cell transplantation in LPS-responsive beige-like anchor (LRBA) deficiency. J Allergy Clin Immunol 2015;135(5):1384–90.e1–8.
50. Albert MH, Gennery AR, Greil J, et al. Successful SCT for Nijmegen breakage syndrome. Bone Marrow Transplant 2010;45(4):622–6.
51. Stray-Pedersen A, Backe PH, Sorte HS, et al. PGM3 mutations cause a congenital disorder of glycosylation with severe immunodeficiency and skeletal dysplasia. Am J Hum Genet 2014;95(1):96–107.
52. Aldave JC, Cachay E, Núñez L, et al. A 1-year-old girl with a gain-of-function STAT1 mutation treated with hematopoietic stem cell transplantation. J Clin Immunol 2013;33(8):1273–5.
53. Milner JD, Vogel TP, Forbes L, et al. Early-onset lymphoproliferation and autoimmunity caused by germline STAT3 gain-of-function mutations. Blood 2015;125(4): 591–9.
54. Kriván G, Erdos M, Kállay K, et al. Successful umbilical cord blood stem cell transplantation in a child with WHIM syndrome. Eur J Haematol 2010;84(3): 274–5.
55. Wehr C, Gennery AR, Lindemans C, et al. Multicenter experience in hematopoietic stem cell transplantation for serious complications of common variable immunodeficiency. J Allergy Clin Immunol 2015;135(4):988–97.e6.
56. Janda A, Sedlacek P, Hönig M, et al. Multicenter survey on the outcome of transplantation of hematopoietic cells in patients with the complete form of DiGeorge anomaly. Blood 2010;116(13):2229–36.
57. Fish JD, Duerst RE, Gelfand EW, et al. Challenges in the use of allogeneic hematopoietic SCT for ectodermal dysplasia with immune deficiency. Bone Marrow Transplant 2009;43(3):217–21.
58. Schimke LF, Rieber N, Rylaarsdam S, et al. A novel gain-of-function IKBA mutation underlies ectodermal dysplasia with immunodeficiency and polyendocrinopathy. J Clin Immunol 2013;33(6):1088–99.
59. Pai SY, Levy O, Jabara HH, et al. Allogeneic transplantation successfully corrects immune defects, but not susceptibility to colitis, in a patient with nuclear factor-kappaB essential modulator deficiency. J Allergy Clin Immunol 2008;122(6): 1113–8.e1.
60. Abu-Arja RF, Chernin LR, Abusin G, et al. Successful hematopoietic cell transplantation in a patient with X-linked agammaglobulinemia and acute myeloid leukemia. Pediatr Blood Cancer 2015;62(9):1674–6.

61. Albert MH, Bittner TC, Nonoyama S, et al. X-linked thrombocytopenia (XLT) due to WAS mutations: clinical characteristics, long-term outcome, and treatment options. Blood 2010;115(16):3231-8.

62. Oshima K, Imai K, Albert MH, et al. Hematopoietic stem cell transplantation for X-linked thrombocytopenia with mutations in the WAS gene. J Clin Immunol 2014;35(1):15-21.

Immunoglobulin Replacement Therapy for Primary Immunodeficiency

 CrossMark

Panida Sriaroon, MD*, Mark Ballow, MD

KEYWORDS

- Immunoglobulin replacement therapy • Intravenous immunoglobulin
- Subcutaneous immunoglobulin • Primary immunodeficiency • IVIG • SCIG

KEY POINTS

- Immunoglobulin replacement therapy helps prevent serious bacterial infections in patients with primary antibody deficiency.
- Dosage adjustment of replacement immunoglobulin must be based on clinical condition and IgG trough or steady-state levels.
- Mild infusion-related reactions are common in intravenous immunoglobulin (IVIG) therapy. Serious systemic reactions from IVIG are rare, and they are even less frequent with subcutaneous immunoglobulin (SCIG).

INTRODUCTION

Over the past 3 decades, IgG has been broadly used as replacement therapy in patients of all ages with primary antibody deficiencies. Successful use of therapeutic IgG to prevent serious infections was first described in 1952 by Bruton[1] in a boy with agammaglobulinemia who had recurrent pneumococcal sepsis. After treatment with monthly injections of immune serum globulin, his gamma globulin levels became detectable and he became free of pneumococcal infections. Shortly afterward, immune serum globulin became the standard treatment for patients with antibody deficiencies who had chronic infection. In the 1950s, IgG was administered via the intramuscular (IM) route, which was associated with pain and risk of nerve injury if large volumes were given in gluteal regions.[2] The IM IgG preparations at that time were not suitable for

Disclosures: None (P. Sriaroon). M. Ballow is receiving an investigator-initiated grant from CSL Behring, and is on the speakers bureau for CSL Behring, Baxter, and Grifols. M. Ballow is on the Advisory Boards for CSL Behring and Baxter. M. Ballow is on the Data Safety Monitoring Board for Kedrion Biopharma, Inc.
Division of Allergy and Immunology, Department of Pediatrics, University of South Florida, 140 7th Avenue South, CRI 4008, Saint Petersburg, FL 33701, USA
* Corresponding author.
E-mail address: psriaroo@health.usf.edu

Immunol Allergy Clin N Am 35 (2015) 713–730
http://dx.doi.org/10.1016/j.iac.2015.07.006
0889-8561/15/$ – see front matter © 2015 Elsevier Inc. All rights reserved.
immunology.theclinics.com

intravenous (IV) use because of severe systemic reactions in up to 25% of patients, particularly in those with antibody deficiencies.[3] In the late 1970s, IVIG, through various modifications of the original Cohn plasma fractionation procedure, became available and gained popularity because of improved tolerability and ability to be infused in high dosages, resulting in prolongation of high serum IgG levels.

At present, there are more than 20 different IgG products commercially available worldwide. Despite having similar biological properties and efficacy, commercial IgG products are manufactured using different methods (**Table 1**) resulting in variations in their physicochemical properties including pH, sodium concentration, osmolality, sodium content, and IgA content. These characteristics may lead to differences in tolerability and adverse events (AEs). Therefore, IgG products are not interchangeable, and brands should not be substituted for each other without physician notification. In the past decade, IgG treatment has evolved to include SCIG, which can be self-administered weekly, or even more frequently, at home and is associated with fewer systemic AEs.[4]

In addition to replacement treatment, IgG has also been used in a wide range of neurologic, autoimmune, and inflammatory conditions because of its immunomodulatory effect when given at high dosage.[5] In this review, the authors provide an overview of IgG therapy for the treatment of patients with primary immunodeficiency disorders (PIDDs), including dosing, route of administration, and various types of AEs. Principles of IgG therapy for PIDD are summarized in **Box 1**. The mechanism of IgG therapy as an immune-modulating agent is beyond the scope of discussion for this article.

CLINICAL APPLICATIONS

For more than 30 years, IgG therapy has been used to treat various immunodeficiency diseases, infections, autoimmune disorders, or inflammatory disorders either at

Table 1
Manufacturing process of IgG preparations

Step	Methods
Gamma globulin acquisition	Cold ethanol fractionation • Cohn method • Cohn-Oncley modification method
Purification (removal of IgG aggregates)	Chromatography • Ion exchange chromatography • Anion chromatography • Caprylate chromatography Enzymatic or chemical modification • Caprylate precipitation, diethylaminoethyl (DEAE) Sephadex • Octanoic acid fractionation/precipitation • Polyethylene glycol precipitation
Additives (stabilization for storage)	Sugars (sucrose, maltose, glucose) Amino acids (proline, glycine)
Viral inactivation/removal	Low pH incubation Treatment at pH 4 plus pepsin Solvent/detergent treatment Caprylate treatment Virus filtration • Depth filtration • Ultrafiltration • Nanofiltration Heat pasteurization

---

Box 1
Principles of IgG therapy for PIDD

IgG is derived from large pools of plasma from 10,000 to 60,000 individuals.

IgG therapy helps prevent serious bacterial infections and long-term infection-related complications, especially pulmonary disease, in patients with PIDD.

Initial dosing is 400 to 600 mg/kg every 4 weeks. Equilibration takes up to 3 months.

Dosage adjustment must be based on clinical condition and IgG trough (IVIG) or steady-state (SCIG) levels. Higher IgG trough levels (>800–1000 mg/dL) may be required in selected patients, especially in those with chronic lung disease.

IVIG products are not interchangeable. Product differences may lead to differences in side effects and tolerability for individual patients.

Mild infusion-rate-related AEs are common in IVIG. Serious systemic AEs from IVIG such as renal failure, thromboembolic events, and hemolysis are rare, and they are even less frequent with SCIG.

SCIG has fewer systemic AEs, whereas local site reactions are common.

IgG antibody-based assays may give false-positive results and should not be used to evaluate patients for infection while they are receiving IgG therapy.

Measles- and varicella-containing vaccines should be delayed 8 to 11 months after receipt of IgG therapy, because immune response to the vaccine may be attenuated.

---

replacement or at immunomodulatory dosages.[5] At present, 8 indications are approved by the US Food and Drug Administration (FDA) for IVIG therapy (**Box 2**), although most usage is off-label.

IgG is largely used to treat patients with PIDD who have impaired antibody production; the passive transfer of antibodies protects against broad categories of infectious pathogens. In patients with significant antibody deficiencies such as congenital agammaglobulinemia and common variable immunodeficiency (CVID), IgG effectively prevents pneumonia and serious bacterial infections[6,7]; the treatment is lifelong for these patients. A short treatment trial of IVIG can be beneficial in selected patients with other partial primary antibody defects such as transient hypogammaglobulinemia of infancy, IgG subclass deficiency, or other PIDD conditions that also have poor specific antibody responses to infectious or immunization agents. In conditions that result in secondary hypogammaglobulinemia such as drug effects, malignancies, or renal or

---

Box 2
FDA-approved uses of IgG therapy

1. Primary immunodeficiency disease or primary antibody immunodeficiency

2. Idiopathic thrombocytopenic purpura

3. Kawasaki disease

4. B-cell chronic lymphocytic leukemia

5. Bone marrow transplant

6. Pediatric human immunodeficiency virus 1 infection

7. Chronic inflammatory demyelinating polyneuropathy

8. Multifocal motor neuropathy

gastrointestinal loss, IgG has not been found to be beneficial except in selected cases.[8]

DOSAGE
Starting Dose

Most practice guidelines recommend a starting dosage of IgG between 400 and 600 mg/kg/month to achieve trough or steady-state IgG levels of approximately 600 to 800 mg/dL. For each 100 mg/kg of IVIG infused, peak serum IgG levels generally increase by 250 mg/dL[9] and trough levels increase by approximately 100 mg/dL.[10] Replacement IgG can be administered in bolus doses every 3 to 4 weeks IV, or the equivalent dose can be divided into daily, weekly, or biweekly subcutaneous (SC) administrations after using the coefficient factor to correct the dose (some use a 1:1 conversion). In some cases, a loading IV dose might be required and may be divided over several days.

Historically, IgG trough levels of greater than 500 mg/dL have been proved to be sufficient to prevent serious bacterial infections.[11] Data from several studies demonstrate that the number and duration of infections and pulmonary outcomes significantly improve when IgG is given at higher doses (600 mg/kg for adults and 800 mg/kg for children) compared with standard doses.[11,12] Some individuals may require higher IgG dosages to maintain a higher serum IgG level, for example, greater than 800 mg/dL, especially in those with very low IgG levels, recurrent pneumonia, or structural lung damage (eg, bronchiectasis).[6] One meta-analysis demonstrated a 5-fold decrease in the incidence of pneumonia in patients whose IgG trough level was 1000 mg/dL versus 500 mg/dL.[13]

Recently, the concept of individualized biological IgG trough level, which is the minimum serum IgG level required to prevent bacterial infections in each individual patient, has been proposed.[14] This level is expected to fall in the age-matched normal reference range but may vary considerably from patient to patient.

The appropriate dosing regimen in obese individuals is not known, because this population has traditionally been excluded from clinical trials. Fixed dosing or dose adjustment according to ideal body weight, rather than actual body weight, has been proposed,[15–17] although it is not used routinely.

Dose Adjustment

Once IgG therapy is initiated, patients must be evaluated for clinical improvement, and the trough or steady-state IgG levels can be measured after 3 months. Once infection rates have improved and IgG levels are in the desirable range, the IgG trough level can be measured every 6 to 12 months. Dose adjustments may be needed in individuals with rapid physical changes, for example, weight gain, pregnancy, or growth spurts after entering puberty. If the patient continues to have significant infections, or IgG trough or steady-state levels remain low, the therapy should be titrated up,[6] which can be accomplished by increasing the dosage or shortening the infusion interval. Patients who experience wear-off effects toward the end of their IVIG dosing cycle often benefit from shortening the infusion interval or switching to SCIG.

ROUTES OF ADMINISTRATION

Therapeutic IgG can be given via IV or SC infusion. The selection of route of administration should be based on the individual patient, the medical status of the patient, and other factors (**Box 3**).[18] Although both routes of administration provide similar efficacy in preventing serious bacterial infections, each offers different advantages and disadvantages (**Table 2**).

> **Box 3**
> **Factors to consider in the selection of administration route**
>
> Availability of IV access
>
> Total monthly dosage
>
> Tolerability of IVIG including headache, myalgias, malaise, and other rate-related side effects
>
> History of serious side effects from IVIG such as aseptic meningitis, thrombosis, or renal failure
>
> Underlying medical conditions that could be relative contraindications to SCIG such as widespread skin disease, limited subcutaneous fat, bleeding disorders, severe thrombocytopenia, and anticoagulation therapy
>
> Patient preference and reliability
>
> Product availability, cost, and access
>
> *Data from* Wasserman RL. Progress in gammaglobulin therapy for immunodeficiency: from subcutaneous to intravenous infusions and back again. J Clin Immunol 2012;32(6):1153–64.

Intravenous Immunoglobulin

One clear advantage of IVIG over SCIG is that it can be infused in a larger volume, therefore the peak level is reached rapidly and the IgG can be given less frequently. The IV route is preferred in patients who need high-dose treatment either during acute infection or for immunomodulating effects. Although newer IVIG preparations are generally associated with fewer infusion-related AEs, because of improved manufacturing methods that remove IgG aggregates, IVIG is still associated with more frequent systemic AEs than SCIG. Because IgG levels can fluctuate substantially during IVIG therapy, with troughs commonly less than half the peak concentration, some patients might experience wear-off effects, such as increased probability of infection or malaise/fatigue, at the end of the dosing cycle owing to serum IgG levels dropping below the protective level.[19]

IVIG manufacturers recommend starting rates of 0.5 to 1 mg/kg/min and increasing gradually up to 3.3 and 8 mg/kg/min. Infusion usually takes 2 to 6 hours when administered at a replacement dosage of 400 to 600 mg/kg per dose. The severity of infusion-related reactions is usually reduced when IVIG is administered at a slower rate, such as 0.5 to 1 mg/kg/min. Higher infusion rates have been associated with more infusion reactions and side effects such as thromboembolic complications. The FDA recommends that infusion rates should be kept at 3 to 4 mg/kg/min in patients who are at risk of renal failure or thrombosis.

IVIG can be administered via peripheral or central IV access. Although some patients need lifelong IgG treatment, a central venous catheter or port placement solely for infusing IVIG is not recommended because of risks such as infection and thrombosis.

Subcutaneous Immunoglobulin

SCIG treatment has grown in popularity during the past decade for several reasons: its efficacy is similar to that of IVIG; it has significantly fewer systemic AEs, shorter infusion time, and almost no wear-off effects; and it offers patients more flexibility in scheduling, a feeling of independence, and improved quality of life.[20–24] After appropriate training, infusion can be administered by the patient or family members at home and while traveling. SCIG might not be a suitable option for elderly patients who lack assistance at home or patients with poor compliance.

Table 2
Comparison of IVIG and SCIG treatment characteristics

	IVIG	SCIG
Administration	IV infusion	SC infusion or rapid push
Infusion frequency	Less frequent, every 3–4 wk	Can be given every day to twice weekly
Volume	Larger	Smaller (minimal change to intravascular volume in high-risk patients)
Time needed	2–6 h	30–90 min (infusion) 5–20 min (push)
High-dose therapy	Possible	Limited by volume tolerated per site and number of sites
IgG level measurement	IgG trough, drawn at the end of 3- to 4-wk infusion cycle	IgG steady state, can be drawn anytime
Pharmacokinetics	Rapid increase in serum level at initiation	—
	Fluctuating serum IgG level	Steady serum IgG level
	Wear-off effects from low trough levels	No wear-off effects
Infusion	Requires IV access	SC infusion; preferred in poor venous access
	Requires trained medical personnel	Can be administered by self, partner, or parent
Infusion location	Hospital, clinic, infusion center, home	Home
Side effects		
Infusion site reactions	Uncommon	Common but usually not serious and tend to decrease over time: swelling, erythema, itching for few hours to few days
Systemic reactions	Common, especially during first few infusions	Uncommon
Patient satisfaction	Preferred by patients not favoring self-administration	Improved quality of life (flexibility, independence, portability)
Cost	Higher (product, IV supplies, facility fee, nursing charges)	Lower (product and infusion supplies, pump)
Patient characteristics	Preferred in patients who are dependent and may be noncompliant	Preferred in patients who are reliable; preferred in patients with renal or cardiac insufficiency

The first SCIG infusion is usually given 1 to 2 weeks after the last IV infusion, as described in most US licensing studies, although some patients who do not have active infections may begin SCIG treatment without transitioning from IVIG. It takes 5 to 12 weeks to achieve a new steady state after switching from IVIG to SCIG, when initiating SCIG in a patient, or making a change in the weekly dosage.[2] This steady-state serum IgG level is generally higher than the serum IgG trough levels observed at the end of IVIG dosing cycle.[4]

The bioavailability of SCIG is approximately 66.7% ± 1.8% of IVIG.[25] At present, in the United States, SCIG prescribing information recommends a 1:1.37 dose adjustment when transitioning from IVIG to SCIG. This figure is based on the FDA requirement in SCIG licensing studies and is extrapolated from the area-under-the-curve calculation, which is the weekly SCIG dose that results in a total serum IgG exposure equivalent to that of the previous IVIG dosage.[26] In the European Union, doses are not routinely adjusted when switching from IVIG to SCIG.[27,28]

Typically, SCIG is administered weekly, but one 20% product was recently approved for administration at variable frequencies, including daily, weekly, or biweekly, providing even more flexible scheduling. SCIG can be administered by gradual infusion or can be rapidly pushed into body sites where there is enough SC fat such as the abdominal wall, inner thigh, posterior upper arm, flanks, or below the buttocks. The infusion is usually given via 1 to 6 sites, depending on the total volume. Administration might take 30 to 90 minutes via infusion pump or 5 to 20 minutes via rapid push, and both methods are practical and well tolerated.[29,30]

A recent development in SCIG therapy is the introduction of a new formulation that uses recombinant human hyaluronidase as a spreading factor. When given with SCIG, hyaluronidase helps increase tissue permeability and facilitates the slow absorption of IgG, thereby allowing SCIG administration in doses (volumes) comparable to IVIG every 3 to 4 weeks.[31] Other improved formulations are in development.

PATIENT MONITORING

To assess treatment response, it is crucial that patients be thoroughly evaluated before initiating IgG therapy to document infection patterns and other comorbidities. Appropriate workup to assess the functional status of a patient's natural antibodies must be conducted, and Ig levels and specific antibodies to prior vaccination should be measured.[32,33] Once IgG treatment is initiated, some IgG-antibody-based tests may give false-positive results because of antibodies in IgG preparations, thus these tests should not be used to measure a patient's antibody function.[34] Therefore, active or past infections in patients receiving IgG therapy should be assessed by using other types of assays that are antigen based, such as the nucleic acid amplification test.

During each infusion, the dosage and lot number should be recorded in case AEs occur. Epinephrine and emergency medications must be available during IVIG infusion, although true anaphylaxis from IgG treatment is extremely rare. All side effects that occur during the infusion should be documented. Follow-up evaluation is recommended at every 3 to 4 months during the first year after IgG treatment initiation and every 6 to 12 months subsequently. The treating physician must review the treatment efficacy and tolerability and measure trough or steady-state IgG serum levels. Complete blood cell count and results of liver and renal function tests should be monitored approximately every 6 months.

Changing the IgG product may occur as a result of poor tolerability or limited product availability, but it is not recommended solely for efficacy reasons. Those who continue to have recurrent or serious infections should have IgG steady-state levels measured and be evaluated to identify reasons for declining efficacy, which may include new comorbidities, persistent infection, IgG loss through gut or kidney, and poor treatment compliance.[35]

ADVERSE EFFECTS

Approximately one-third of patients receiving IVIG experience systemic AEs during or within 72 hours after infusions. Most reactions are benign and can be managed easily, whereas some reactions can be more serious or lead to long-term complications (**Table 3**). Nearly all infusion-related reactions are the result of components in the IgG products, rapid infusion rate, patient's risk factors, or combinations thereof (**Box 4**).

Table 3
Adverse effects of IgG therapy

System	Common	Rare
Constitutional or systemic	Fever, chills, fatigue, malaise, flushing, chills, anorexia, musculoskeletal pain, myalgia, arthralgia, joint swelling, flulike symptoms, anaphylactoid reactions, hypothermia	Full-blown anaphylaxis
Neurologic	Headache, migraine, anxiety, dizziness	Aseptic meningitis, diffuse pain, dysesthesia, weakness, progressive neurodegeneration
Respiratory	Dyspnea, cough, bronchospasm	Pleural effusion, transfusion-related acute lung injury
Cardiovascular	Hypertension, hypotension, tachycardia, palpitation, chest pain	Arrhythmia, myocardial infarction, shock
Gastrointestinal	Nausea, vomiting, cramping, diarrhea	—
Renal	—	Hyponatremia, tubular damage, acute renal failure
Cutaneous	Urticaria, nonspecific maculopapular rash, pruritus, tingling sensation	Erythema multiforme, vasculitis
Hematologic	Hemolysis (not clinically significant), positive result of direct Coombs test	Thromboembolic events (deep vein thrombosis, stroke), hyperviscosity, neutropenia, coagulopathy
Others	—	Blood-borne infections, uveitis, alopecia, serum sickness

Adapted from Bonilla FA. Intravenous immunoglobulin: adverse reactions and management. J Allergy Clin Immunol 2008;122(6):1239; with permission.

Acute Systemic Adverse Events During or Immediately After Immunoglobulin G Infusions

Acute systemic AEs during IVIG infusion are common, often benign and reversible, and usually related to the infusion rate. The most common side effect is headache[34]; other symptoms include low-grade temperature, chills, flushing, nausea, fatigue, myalgia, tachycardia, chest tightness, and musculoskeletal pain. Rarely, patients experience more serious reactions such as dyspnea, vomiting, hypotension, or hypertension. Although acute systemic AEs usually accompany or occur immediately after IgG infusions, some reactions such as headache, fatigue, and myalgia may be delayed and in some patients, may last several hours or days after the infusion.[36]

These infusion-related reactions are typically due to the IgG aggregates that are formed during infusion and their complement-fixing activity.[37] These antibodies can form oligomeric or polymeric IgG complexes that can interact with Fc receptors on phagocytes and monocytes and trigger the release of inflammatory mediators through complement activation. Newer liquid IVIG preparations are generally better tolerated and associated with fewer and less-severe reactions. This improvement is because of developments in manufacturing technologies, especially the advances in liquid formulation and the addition of stabilizers to prevent IgG complex formation.

Box 4
Risk factors for adverse effects from IgG therapy

Product related

Type of stabilizer

IgA content

Product with prior history of infusion reaction

Osmolality

Sodium content

Procoagulants

Vasoactive enzymes; kallikreins

Isohemagglutinin (anti-A, anti-B, anti-D, anti-Kell)

Procoagulant coagulation factors (factors XI and XIa)

Infusion related

First infusion (at initiation or after a long break)

Large dose

Rapid infusion rate

No preinfusion or postinfusion hydration

Patient related

Advanced age

Active infection or fever at the time of infusion

Prior history of infusion reaction

Hypercoagulable state

Permanent indwelling venous catheter

Prior thrombosis

Cardiovascular risk factors (hypertension, dyslipidemia, diabetes, and smoking)

Preexisting renal disease (especially diabetes and older age)

These infusion-related AEs occur most commonly during the first few infusions and in patients with more profound hypogammaglobulinemia who are naive to IgG treatment or have had interruptions in the IgG treatment. In addition, patients with active infections seem to have more severe reactions; this is believed to be the result of antigen-antibody complex formation during the infusion or the rapid release of lipopolysaccharide or other components of pathogens already present in the recipient.[34] The risk of reactions also increases when patients already on IgG treatment are given a different IVIG product.[38] Data from one licensing study showed that up to 20% of patients had AEs during or within 72 hours after the first infusion of a new IVIG product and that the reactions reduced to 16% after the second, 6% after the third, and only 2% after the fourth infusion.[39] The reason for this is not known.

There are several measures for management and prevention of mild IV infusion-related reactions such as headache, myalgia, and fatigue. When these symptoms occur during IVIG treatment, slowing the infusion rate or briefly discontinuing the infusion is usually effective. Symptoms are often relieved by treatment with acetaminophen or ibuprofen, and diphenhydramine. Severe headaches may be treated with systemic corticosteroids alone or in combination with ibuprofen or antimigraine medication such as 5-hydroxytryptamine receptor antagonists.[40] Some patients might require treatment for as long as 72 hours after the infusion is completed.[41]

In patients with frequent reactions, premedication before infusion and a slow infusion rate have been proved effective in preventing AEs.[10,37,42] Infusion rate should be started at 0.5 to 1 mg/kg/min and gradually increased as tolerated and not exceed 8 mg/kg/min. If side effects continue despite prophylactic measures, changing the IVIG product or switching to SCIG should be considered. However, the decision must be made carefully because systemic AEs can also occur with new brands.[39] In patients requiring large doses of IgG, fractionated dosing over several days is helpful in preventing reactions.

Anaphylaxis Versus Anaphylactoid Reactions

True IgE-mediated anaphylactic reactions to IVIG products are uncommon.[43] In contrast, anaphylactoid reactions may occur as a result of more severe reactions to IgG aggregates. These reactions often decrease in severity over time with repeated use of the same IVIG product and are usually associated with hypertension, in contrast to IgE-mediated anaphylaxis, which is commonly associated with hypotension. Severe anaphylactoid reactions predominantly involve activation of the complement and the kallikrein-kinin systems, resulting in release of cytokines and lipid mediators.[34] These reactions are usually seen in patients receiving IVIG who also have active infections. Therefore, patients with active infections should be afebrile and actively treated with antibiotics before receiving IVIG therapy.

Reactions Due to Anti-immunoglobulin A Antibodies

The presence of preformed IgE or IgG antibodies to IgA can cause severe reactions including anaphylaxis, in patients with hypogammaglobulinemia and absent serum IgA who are receiving IgA-containing IgG or blood products.[44–46] True anaphylaxis due to IgE anti-IgA is extremely rare and has been reported in only a few cases.[44] Up to a third of immunodeficient subjects with absent serum IgA have been found to have IgG anti-IgA, but only a fraction experience anaphylaxis.[44]

The risk of reactions to IVIG varies among immunodeficient patients with low serum IgA levels. Patients with CVID and undetectable levels of serum IgA (<5 mg/dL or <7 mg/dL) are at highest risk. Patients with profound hypogammaglobulinemia, agammaglobulinemia (such as X-linked agammaglobulinemia), and low, but detectable serum IgA levels are presumably not at risk for anaphylaxis from IVIG. Regardless, caution should be used when administering IVIG products in individuals with absent serum IgA levels. IVIG infusion should be initiated slowly at 0.001 mL/kg/min, and the rate can be increased gradually with subsequent infusions. Anti-IgA antibody levels are not routinely measured in clinical practice owing to their limited availability, and their predictive value is not known.[44]

All currently available IVIG preparations have at least trace amounts of IgA, which range widely from less than or equal to 2 to greater than 700 µg/mL. If anaphylaxis occurs, the product must be changed to one with the lowest IgA content (preferably ≤25 µg/mL) or SCIG should be considered. In general, systemic reactions to SCIG are uncommon, and SCIG has been used successfully in patients with PIDD who have reacted previously to IgA-containing IVIG.[40,44,46–49]

Aseptic Meningitis

Aseptic meningitis, characterized by severe, prolonged headache; photophobia; stiff neck; and cerebrospinal fluid (CSF) pleocytosis, is a slightly more serious side effect to

IVIG, which seldom leads to long-term complications.[50] Aseptic meningitis usually is associated with high-dose IVIG (1–2 g/kg) and rapid infusion, especially in the treatment of autoimmune or inflammatory conditions[41,50–52]; it is rarely seen in patients with PIDD.[42] Symptoms often begin within 24 hours after infusion and may last several days. The cause remains unclear, but migraine has been described as a risk factor.[41] It has been suggested that meningeal irritation may be caused by IgG from IVIG and/or immune complexes of therapeutic IgG and endogenous IgG in the CSF.[53] Treatment with corticosteroids such as prednisone or hydrocortisone for a few days may be effective.

Renal Complications

Acute renal insufficiency and/or failure is a rare but serious AE to IgG replacement therapy.[54] The mechanisms of renal injury from IVIG may involve osmotic injury to the proximal renal tubular cells.[55] Acute renal damage has primarily been associated with preparations that contain sucrose as the stabilizer, although reactions to preparations that contain other sugars or amino acids have also been reported.[56] Clinical presentation can range from asymptomatic increases in serum urea nitrogen and creatinine levels to full-blown renal failure. Although most cases respond well to conservative treatment within 4 to 10 days after IVIG is discontinued, permanent renal failure and mortality have been described, especially in cases with serious underlying conditions.[56] Risk factors include preexisting renal disease, diabetes, advanced age (>65 years), paraproteinemia, dehydration, sepsis, and concomitant use of nephrotoxic agents. Over half of the reported cases were in patients who were treated for idiopathic thrombocytopenic purpura, which may be related to the higher IVIG dose, while less than 5% were reported in patients treated for PIDD.

It is recommended that the infusion rate for sucrose-containing products should not exceed 3 mg/kg/min. Patients with underlying renal disease should use a non–sucrose-containing product, and IVIG solutions more concentrated than 5% should be avoided. Prehydrating IV fluid and fractionating doses into smaller ones given on different days may be beneficial in preventing renal complications.

Acute Hemolysis and Hemolytic Anemia

Hemolytic reactions are a rare but serious complication of IgG therapy. The reactions likely occur as a result of passive transfer of anti-A or anti-B IgG isohemagglutinins in gamma globulin products.[57] As type O is the most common human blood type, it is likely that anti-A and anti-B antibodies can be found at significant amounts in the commercial IgG preparations. The major risk factors are infusion of large doses, active systemic inflammatory state (suggested by elevated levels of inflammatory markers), and non-O blood group. There are case reports of reactions in patients with blood type O, suggesting that other non-A/B antibodies might also contribute.[58–60] Although rare, there are still cases of hemolysis, even though all current IgG preparations licensed in the European Union and the United States are required to contain less than or equal to 1:64 anti-A to anti-B titers in a direct hemagglutinin assay.[61–63]

The presentations range from positive results of Coombs test in the absence of symptoms to clinically significant or even severe intravascular hemolysis requiring blood transfusion, which was reported almost exclusively in patients receiving high doses of IVIG for immunomodulatory purposes.[57–60,64–66] Acute renal failure and deaths have also been described. In patients at high risk, the IgG treatment should be fractionated into several small doses given on different days. Changing to a different IVIG product may be helpful, but reactions may still occur. Acute hemolysis is rarely seen in patients receiving replacement IVIG for PIDD (0.4–0.8 g/kg) based on data from several licensing studies.[34] Hemolysis has been described in patients receiving SCIG but less frequently.

Thromboembolic Events

Wide ranges of thrombotic complications have been reported since therapeutic IgG was introduced, including local thromboses at infusion sites, deep vein thrombosis, myocardial infarction, pulmonary embolism, transient ischemic attacks, stroke, and transfusion-related acute lung injury.[34,67–69] Although the true incidence is not known, thromboembolic events (TEEs) have been estimated in less than 0.01% to 1% of patients receiving IgG treatment.[57] Potential risk factors for this AE are broad and include advanced age, male gender, smoking, prolonged immobilization, previous history of venous or arterial thrombosis, diabetes, dyslipidemia, anemia, polycythemia, hypercoagulable state, hyperviscosity, supplemental estrogens, indwelling vascular catheters and cardiovascular risk factors such as hypertension, atrial fibrillation, and coronary artery disease.[47,70] TEEs can still occur in patients with no known risk factors and following IgG administration by any route: IM, IV, or SC.[34] TEEs are likely due to increased serum viscosity from the IgG itself[71] and/or hypertonic state (caused by sugars or other stabilizers) that may induce platelet activation.[71–73] First infusions, large dose, and rapid infusion rate are also associated with TEEs.[57]

Measures to reduce risks for developing TEEs include slow infusion rate (0.05 g/kg/h for the first hour and 0.1 g/kg/h thereafter), preinfusion/postinfusion hydration, and limiting IVIG administration to 0.4 to 0.5 g/kg/d.[47] Prescribers should consider fractionating IVIG doses to be given on consecutive days if a larger dose is needed. In high-risk patients, prophylaxis with aspirin, antiplatelet medication, or low-molecular-weight heparin may be required.

Recently, activated factor XI (FXIa) has been identified as the probable procoagulant contaminant that causes thromboembolic complications in some IgG products.[74,75] Investigation of a withdrawn IVIG product shows that FXIa activity was increased in the product, likely a result of slight changes in manufacturing procedures. The increase in FXIa likely correlates with the rates of TEEs, although the complications are rarely seen with products with low FXIa levels.[57] Therefore, it is likely that patients' individual risk factors also play a role. The discovery that factor XI (FXI)/FXIa from IVIG products can cause TEEs has led to changes in manufacturing processes for IVIG such as the use of high-sensitivity thrombin-generation assays to measure the thrombogenic potential of IgG and the use of newer chromatographic purification procedures and immunoadsorbents of FXI/FXIa.[76]

Infectious Complications

IVIG is considered a pooled blood product and therefore poses risks of blood-borne pathogen transmission. Bacterial particles are considerably larger than other infectious pathogens and therefore can be effectively removed with simple filtration techniques during the manufacturing process. In contrast, viral and prion particles can be difficult to remove. In the 1990s, there were cases of hepatitis C virus (HCV) infection reported in patients receiving experimental lots of IVIG products in the United States and Europe. Consequently, viral inactivation steps have been added to the manufacturing procedures, which have resulted in markedly decreased risk of HCV and other viral transmission. Standard procedures to reduce risk of infectious disease transmission include donor screening for viruses and several viral inactivation and removal steps, which result in the potential removal of 10 to 20 $\log_{10}$ reduction values of viral particles.[36,77] At present, IgG products are considered to be free of infectious pathogens, and there has not been a confirmed case of human immunodeficiency virus transmission from IgG treatment.

Reactions to Subcutaneous Immunoglobulin

One major advantage of SCIG over IVIG therapy is the rarity of systemic AEs, which are reported to occur in fewer than 5% of patients.[78–81] Berger[82] analyzed data from several studies that included over 40,000 SCIG infusions and showed that the overall incidence of systemic AEs was only 0.43%; this is likely due to the smaller doses administered at each administration and the relatively gradual systemic absorption of SCIG. In contrast, local site reactions such as itchiness, swelling, warmth, redness, induration, soreness, or bruising are common, occurring in up to 75% of patients.[79–81] The swelling is a result of the infused IgG product volume (20–30 mL per site) being administered into SC tissue over a short period and additional fluid drawn into the site because of osmotic difference. The redness, warmth, and itching are likely due to locally produced inflammatory mediators, which enhance vascular permeability.[4,83] Symptoms generally last for less than 24 to 48 hours and do not require treatment. In most cases, the severity and frequency of local reactions lessen over time with continued SCIG therapy and do not usually lead to treatment discontinuation.[78] Long-term sequelae at the infusion sites such as fibrosis, atrophy, lipodystrophy, or SC nodules have not been described.[34]

SUMMARY

IgG replacement is critical in the treatment of many PIDDs that affect antibody production, and in recent years, its use has expanded to include other autoimmune and inflammatory disorders. The number of indications for IgG therapy is steadily increasing. Clinicians must be familiar with differences among products and AEs or other complications that might occur from IgG treatment; this will help to ensure that they select the appropriate treatment options for individual patients. Considerations include route of administration, dosage, interval, infusion rates, and treatment duration. Dosage adjustments must be based on clinical outcomes and the IgG trough or steady-state levels, especially in patients with chronic lung disease.

As lifelong IgG replacement is the only therapy available to most patients with primary antibody deficiency, prescribers should take a thorough history and identify risk factors before developing a treatment regimen. Patients should be evaluated for risk factors and should be monitored closely during and after IgG infusions. Moreover, patients should be educated about potential AEs and treatment expectations. Success depends on several factors, including long-term follow-up, regular monitoring, and interaction between patients and multidisciplinary teams.

Several manufacturers are refining purification steps to make IgG products safer, better tolerated, more concentrated, and consequently easier and less expensive to administer. Many of these efforts have produced products that can be safely infused IV in the home setting or can be given SC by patients and their family members. The new formulation using recombinant human hyaluronidase, which allows more rapid infusions of larger IgG volumes by the SC route, is already approved in the United States and European Union. New formulations and infusion devices are being developed, which will likely improve patients' quality of life.

ACKNOWLEDGMENTS

The authors thank Dr Jane Carver for reviewing this article.

REFERENCES

1. Bruton OC. Agammaglobulinemia. Pediatrics 1952;9(6):722–8.
2. Lieberman P, Berger M. Intramuscular versus intravenous immunoglobulin replacement therapy and measurement of immunoglobulin levels during immunoglobulin replacement therapy. J Allergy Clin Immunol 2013;1(6):705–6.
3. Eibl MM. History of immunoglobulin replacement. Immunol Allergy Clin North Am 2008;28(4):737–64, viii.
4. Berger M. Subcutaneous administration of IgG. Immunol Allergy Clin North Am 2008;28(4):779–802, viii.
5. Orange JS, Hossny EM, Weiler CR, et al. Use of intravenous immunoglobulin in human disease: a review of evidence by members of the Primary Immunodeficiency Committee of the American Academy of Allergy, Asthma and Immunology. J Allergy Clin Immunol 2006;117(4 Suppl):S525–53.
6. Lucas M, Lee M, Lortan J, et al. Infection outcomes in patients with common variable immunodeficiency disorders: relationship to immunoglobulin therapy over 22 years. J Allergy Clin Immunol 2010;125(6):1354–60.e4.
7. Albin S, Cunningham-Rundles C. An update on the use of immunoglobulin for the treatment of immunodeficiency disorders. Immunotherapy 2014;6(10):1113–26.
8. Compagno N, Malipiero G, Cinetto F, et al. Immunoglobulin replacement therapy in secondary hypogammaglobulinemia. Front Immunol 2014;5:626.
9. Ochs HD, Fischer SH, Wedgwood RJ, et al. Comparison of high-dose and low-dose intravenous immunoglobulin therapy in patients with primary immunodeficiency diseases. Am J Med 1984;76(3A):78–82.
10. Stiehm E. Immunodeficiency disorders general conditions. 4th edition. Philadelphia (PA): Saunders; 1996.
11. Roifman CM, Levison H, Gelfand EW. High-dose versus low-dose intravenous immunoglobulin in hypogammaglobulinaemia and chronic lung disease. Lancet 1987;1(8541):1075–7.
12. Eijkhout HW, van Der Meer JW, Kallenberg CG, et al. The effect of two different dosages of intravenous immunoglobulin on the incidence of recurrent infections in patients with primary hypogammaglobulinemia. A randomized, double-blind, multicenter crossover trial. Ann Intern Med 2001;135(3):165–74.
13. Orange JS, Grossman WJ, Navickis RJ, et al. Impact of trough IgG on pneumonia incidence in primary immunodeficiency: a meta-analysis of clinical studies. Clin Immunol 2010;137(1):21–30.
14. Bonagura VR. Illustrative cases on individualizing immunoglobulin therapy in primary immunodeficiency disease. Ann Allergy Asthma Immunol 2013;111(6 Suppl):S10–3.
15. Khan S, Grimbacher B, Boecking C, et al. Serum trough IgG level and annual intravenous immunoglobulin dose are not related to body size in patients on regular replacement therapy. Drug Metab Lett 2011;5(2):132–6.
16. Rocchio MA, Hussey AP, Southard RA, et al. Impact of ideal body weight dosing for all inpatient i.v. immune globulin indications. Am J Health Syst Pharm 2013;70(9):751–2.
17. Siegel J. Immunoglobulins and obesity: dosing. Considerations Pharmay Pract News 2013;2013:40. Available at: http://pharmacypracticenews.com/ViewArticle.aspx?d=Clinical&d_id=50&i=August+2013&i_id=985&a_id=23771. Accessed April 9, 2015.
18. Wasserman RL. Progress in gammaglobulin therapy for immunodeficiency: from subcutaneous to intravenous infusions and back again. J Clin Immunol 2012;32(6):1153–64.

19. Misbah SA. Effective dosing strategies for therapeutic immunoglobulin: managing wear-off effects in antibody replacement to immunomodulation. Clin Exp Immunol 2014;178(Suppl 1):70–1.
20. Gardulf A, Hammarstrom L, Smith CI. Home treatment of hypogammaglobulinaemia with subcutaneous gammaglobulin by rapid infusion. Lancet 1991; 338(8760):162–6.
21. Abrahamsen TG, Sandersen H, Bustnes A. Home therapy with subcutaneous immunoglobulin infusions in children with congenital immunodeficiencies. Pediatrics 1996;98(6 Pt 1):1127–31.
22. Thomas MJ, Brennan VM, Chapel HH. Rapid subcutaneous immunoglobulin infusions in children. Lancet 1993;342(8884):1432–3.
23. Gaspar J, Gerritsen B, Jones A. Immunoglobulin replacement treatment by rapid subcutaneous infusion. Arch Dis Child 1998;79(1):48–51.
24. Abolhassani H, Sadaghiani MS, Aghamohammadi A, et al. Home-based subcutaneous immunoglobulin versus hospital-based intravenous immunoglobulin in treatment of primary antibody deficiencies: systematic review and meta analysis. J Clin Immunol 2012;32(6):1180–92.
25. Berger M, Jolles S, Orange JS, et al. Bioavailability of IgG administered by the subcutaneous route. J Clin Immunol 2013;33(5):984–90.
26. Berger M, Rojavin M, Kiessling P, et al. Pharmacokinetics of subcutaneous immunoglobulin and their use in dosing of replacement therapy in patients with primary immunodeficiencies. Clin Immunol 2011;139(2):133–41.
27. Jolles S, Bernatowska E, de Gracia J, et al. Efficacy and safety of Hizentra((R)) in patients with primary immunodeficiency after a dose-equivalent switch from intravenous or subcutaneous replacement therapy. Clin Immunol 2011;141(1): 90–102.
28. Gardulf A, Nicolay U, Asensio O, et al. Rapid subcutaneous IgG replacement therapy is effective and safe in children and adults with primary immunodeficiencies–a prospective, multi-national study. J Clin Immunol 2006;26(2): 177–85.
29. Shapiro RS. Subcutaneous immunoglobulin therapy given by subcutaneous rapid push vs infusion pump: a retrospective analysis. Ann Allergy Asthma Immunol 2013;111(1):51–5.
30. Shapiro RS. Subcutaneous immunoglobulin: rapid push vs infusion pump in pediatrics. Pediatr Allergy Immunol 2013;24(1):49–53.
31. Wasserman RL, Melamed I, Stein MR, et al. Recombinant human hyaluronidase-facilitated subcutaneous infusion of human immunoglobulins for primary immunodeficiency. J Allergy Clin Immunol 2012;130(4):951–7.e11.
32. Bonilla FA, Bernstein IL, Khan DA, et al. Practice parameter for the diagnosis and management of primary immunodeficiency. Ann Allergy Asthma Immunol 2005; 94(5 Suppl 1):S1–63.
33. Orange JS, Ballow M, Stiehm ER, et al. Use and interpretation of diagnostic vaccination in primary immunodeficiency: a working group report of the Basic and Clinical Immunology Interest Section of the American Academy of Allergy, Asthma & Immunology. J Allergy Clin Immunol 2012;130(3 Suppl):S1–24.
34. Berger M. Adverse effects of IgG therapy. J Allergy Clin Immunol 2013;1(6): 558–66.
35. Peter JG, Chapel H. Immunoglobulin replacement therapy for primary immunodeficiencies. Immunotherapy 2014;6(7):853–69.
36. Ballow M. Safety of IGIV therapy and infusion-related adverse events. Immunol Res 2007;38(1–3):122–32.

37. Lederman HM, Roifman CM, Lavi S, et al. Corticosteroids for prevention of adverse reactions to intravenous immune serum globulin infusions in hypogammaglobulinemic patients. Am J Med 1986;81(3):443–6.

38. Ballow M. Clinical and investigational considerations for the use of IGIV therapy. Am J Health Syst Pharm 2005;62(16 Suppl 3):S12–8 [quiz: S19–21].

39. Berger M, Pinciaro PJ, Flebogamma I. Safety, efficacy, and pharmacokinetics of Flebogamma 5% [immune globulin intravenous (human)] for replacement therapy in primary immunodeficiency diseases. J Clin Immunol 2004;24(4): 389–96.

40. Finkel AG, Howard JF Jr, Mann JD. Successful treatment of headache related to intravenous immunoglobulin with antimigraine medications. Headache 1998; 38(4):317–21.

41. Sekul EA, Cupler EJ, Dalakas MC. Aseptic meningitis associated with high-dose intravenous immunoglobulin therapy: frequency and risk factors. Ann Intern Med 1994;121(4):259–62.

42. Roberton DM, Hosking CS. Use of methylprednisolone as prophylaxis for immediate adverse infusion reactions in hypogammaglobulinaemic patients receiving intravenous immunoglobulin: a controlled trial. Aust Paediatr J 1988;24(3):174–7.

43. Brennan VM, Salome-Bentley NJ, Chapel HM, et al. Prospective audit of adverse reactions occurring in 459 primary antibody-deficient patients receiving intravenous immunoglobulin. Clin Exp Immunol 2003;133(2):247–51.

44. Rachid R, Bonilla FA. The role of anti-IgA antibodies in causing adverse reactions to gamma globulin infusion in immunodeficient patients: a comprehensive review of the literature. J Allergy Clin Immunol 2012;129(3):628–34.

45. Burks AW, Sampson HA, Buckley RH. Anaphylactic reactions after gamma globulin administration in patients with hypogammaglobulinemia. Detection of IgE antibodies to IgA. N Engl J Med 1986;314(9):560–4.

46. Bjorkander J, Hammarstrom L, Smith CI, et al. Immunoglobulin prophylaxis in patients with antibody deficiency syndromes and anti-IgA antibodies. J Clin Immunol 1987;7(1):8–15.

47. Stiehm ER. Adverse effects of human immunoglobulin therapy. Transfus Med Rev 2013;27(3):171–8.

48. Eijkhout HW, van den Broek PJ, van der Meer JW. Substitution therapy in immunodeficient patients with anti-IgA antibodies or severe adverse reactions to previous immunoglobulin therapy. Neth J Med 2003;61(6):213–7.

49. Sundin U, Nava S, Hammarstrom L. Induction of unresponsiveness against IgA in IgA-deficient patients on subcutaneous immunoglobulin infusion therapy. Clin Exp Immunol 1998;112(2):341–6.

50. Brannagan TH 3rd, Nagle KJ, Lange DJ, et al. Complications of intravenous immune globulin treatment in neurologic disease. Neurology 1996;47(3):674–7.

51. Scribner CL, Kapit RM, Phillips ET, et al. Aseptic meningitis and intravenous immunoglobulin therapy. Ann Intern Med 1994;121(4):305–6.

52. Kato E, Shindo S, Eto Y, et al. Administration of immune globulin associated with aseptic meningitis. JAMA 1988;259(22):3269–71.

53. Mathy I, Gille M, Van Raemdonck F, et al. Neurological complications of intravenous immunoglobulin (IVIg) therapy: an illustrative case of acute encephalopathy following IVIg therapy and a review of the literature. Acta Neurol Belg 1998;98(4): 347–51.

54. Cantu TG, Hoehn-Saric EW, Burgess KM, et al. Acute renal failure associated with immunoglobulin therapy. Am J kidney Dis 1995;25(2):228–34.

55. Zhang R, Szerlip HM. Reemergence of sucrose nephropathy: acute renal failure caused by high-dose intravenous immune globulin therapy. South Med J 2000; 93(9):901–4.
56. Centers for Disease Control and Prevention (CDC). Renal insufficiency and failure associated with immune globulin intravenous therapy–United States, 1985–1998. MMWR Morb Mortal Wkly Rep 1999;48(24):518–21.
57. Bonilla FA. Adverse effects of immunoglobulin G therapy: thromboembolism and haemolysis. Clin Exp Immunol 2014;178(Suppl 1):72–4.
58. Daw Z, Padmore R, Neurath D, et al. Hemolytic transfusion reactions after administration of intravenous immune (gamma) globulin: a case series analysis. Transfusion 2008;48(8):1598–601.
59. Kahwaji J, Barker E, Pepkowitz S, et al. Acute hemolysis after high-dose intravenous immunoglobulin therapy in highly HLA sensitized patients. Clin J Am Soc Nephrol 2009;4(12):1993–7.
60. Morgan S, Sorensen P, Vercellotti G, et al. Haemolysis after treatment with intravenous immunoglobulin due to anti-A. Transfus Med 2011;21(4):267–70.
61. Bellac CL, Polatti D, Hottiger T, et al. Anti-A and anti-B haemagglutinin levels in intravenous immunoglobulins: are they on the rise? A comparison of four different analysis methods and six products. Biologicals 2014;42(1):57–64.
62. Welles CC, Tambra S, Lafayette RA. Hemoglobinuria and acute kidney injury requiring hemodialysis following intravenous immunoglobulin infusion. Am J kidney Dis 2010;55(1):148–51.
63. Strategies to address hemolytic complications of immune globulin infusions. Workshop on Risk Mitigation Measure Strategies. 2014. Available at: http://www.fda.gov/downloads/BiologicsBloodVaccines/NewsEvents/WorkshopsMeetings Conferences/UCM387078.pdf. Accessed April 9, 2015.
64. Robertson VM, Dickson LG, Romond EH, et al. Positive antiglobulin tests due to intravenous immunoglobulin in patients who received bone marrow transplant. Transfusion 1987;27(1):28–31.
65. Wilson JR, Bhoopalam H, Fisher M. Hemolytic anemia associated with intravenous immunoglobulin. Muscle Nerve 1997;20(9):1142–5.
66. Pintova S, Bhardwaj AS, Aledort LM. IVIG–a hemolytic culprit. N Engl J Med 2012; 367(10):974–6.
67. Caress JB, Hobson-Webb L, Passmore LV, et al. Case-control study of thromboembolic events associated with IV immunoglobulin. J Neurol 2009;256(3):339–42.
68. Caress JB, Cartwright MS, Donofrio PD, et al. The clinical features of 16 cases of stroke associated with administration of IVIg. Neurology 2003;60(11):1822–4.
69. Go RS, Call TG. Deep venous thrombosis of the arm after intravenous immunoglobulin infusion: case report and literature review of intravenous immunoglobulin-related thrombotic complications. Mayo Clin Proc 2000;75(1): 83–5.
70. Rajabally YA, Kearney DA. Thromboembolic complications of intravenous immunoglobulin therapy in patients with neuropathy: a two-year study. J Neurol Sci 2011;308(1–2):124–7.
71. Reinhart WH, Berchtold PE. Effect of high-dose intravenous immunoglobulin therapy on blood rheology. Lancet 1992;339(8794):662–4.
72. Dalakas MC. High-dose intravenous immunoglobulin and serum viscosity: risk of precipitating thromboembolic events. Neurology 1994;44(2):223–6.
73. Crouch ED, Watson LE. Intravenous immunoglobulin-related acute coronary syndrome and coronary angiography in idiopathic thrombocytopenic purpura–a case report and literature review. Angiology 2002;53(1):113–7.

74. FDA Safety Communication: Updated information on the risks of thrombosis and hemolysis potentially related to administration of intravenous, subcutaneous and intramuscular human immune globulin products. 2012. Available at: http://www.fda.gov/biologicsbloodvaccines/safetyavailability/ucm327934.htm. Accessed April 9, 2015.

75. Ovanesov MV. Laboratory investigation that identified the cause of thromboembolic events in patients receiving immunoglobulin treatments. 2012. Available at: http://www.fda.gov/downloads/AdvisoryCommittees/CommitteesMeetingMaterials/ScienceBoardtotheFoodandDrugAdministration/UCM321916.pdf. Accessed April 9, 2015.

76. Roemisch J, Kaar W, Zoechling A, et al. Identification of activated FXI as the major biochemical root cause in IVIG batches associated with thromboembolic events. Analytical and experimental approaches resulting in corrective and preventive measures implemented into the Octagam manufacturing process. WebmedCentral IMMUNOTHERAPY. 2011;2(6). Available at: http://www.webmedcentral.com/article_view/2002. Accessed April 9, 2015.

77. Ballow M. Intravenous immunoglobulins: clinical experience and viral safety. J Am Pharm Assoc 2002;42(3):449–58 [quiz: 458–9].

78. Ochs HD, Gupta S, Kiessling P, et al, Subcutaneous IgG Study Group. Safety and efficacy of self-administered subcutaneous immunoglobulin in patients with primary immunodeficiency diseases. J Clin Immunol 2006;26(3):265–73.

79. Hagan JB, Fasano MB, Spector S, et al. Efficacy and safety of a new 20% immunoglobulin preparation for subcutaneous administration, IgPro20, in patients with primary immunodeficiency. J Clin Immunol 2010;30(5):734–45.

80. Wasserman RL, Irani AM, Tracy J, et al. Pharmacokinetics and safety of subcutaneous immune globulin (human), 10% caprylate/chromatography purified in patients with primary immunodeficiency disease. Clin Exp Immunol 2010;161(3):518–26.

81. Wasserman RL, Melamed I, Kobrynski L, et al. Efficacy, safety, and pharmacokinetics of a 10% liquid immune globulin preparation (GAMMAGARD LIQUID, 10%) administered subcutaneously in subjects with primary immunodeficiency disease. J Clin Immunol 2011;31(3):323–31.

82. Berger M. Subcutaneous immunoglobulin replacement in primary immunodeficiencies. Clin Immunol 2004;112(1):1–7.

83. Wasserman RL. Common infusion-related reactions to subcutaneous immunoglobulin therapy: managing patient expectations. Patient Prefer Adherence 2008;2:163–6.

Autoimmune Disease in Primary Immunodeficiency

At the Crossroads of Anti-Infective Immunity and Self-Tolerance

Maryam Saifi, MD, Christian A. Wysocki, MD, PhD*

KEYWORDS

- Primary immunodeficiency • Autoimmunity • Tolerance • Regulatory T cell
- Apoptosis • Common variable immunodeficiency

KEY POINTS

- Identification of gene defects in primary immunodeficiencies complicated by autoimmune diseases has expanded the understanding of central and peripheral self-tolerance.
- This knowledge is in turn expanding the understanding of more complex, polygenic diseases of immunodeficiency and immune dysregulation, such as common variable immunodeficiency (CVID).
- Certain gene mutations, resulting in autoimmune phenotypes with incomplete penetrance, may act as disease modifiers in complex diseases, such as CVID, increasing predisposition toward autoimmunity.

INTRODUCTION

Autoimmunity and primary immunodeficiency (PID) are frequently associated. This seemingly paradoxic relationship highlights the inherent mechanistic links between proper development of the various elements of the immune system, and the selection and regulatory mechanisms that maintain self-tolerance. Here, various immunologic syndromes are discussed in which this paradoxic relationship occurs, and the lesions in self-tolerance and immunoregulation are systematically explored that contribute to autoimmunity in these diseases. The authors have tried to be comprehensive, but, because this topic is broad, certain immunologic syndromes, such as the autoinflammatory syndromes (periodic fever syndromes), were thought to fall outside the scope

Disclaimers: None.
Division of Allergy and Immunology, Department of Internal Medicine, UT Southwestern Medical Center, 5323 Harry Hines Boulevard, Dallas, TX 75390-8859, USA
* Corresponding author.
E-mail address: Christian.Wysocki@utsouthwestern.edu

Immunol Allergy Clin N Am 35 (2015) 731–752
http://dx.doi.org/10.1016/j.iac.2015.07.007
0889-8561/15/$ – see front matter © 2015 Elsevier Inc. All rights reserved.

of this review and have been reviewed elsewhere.[1] For defective tolerance mechanisms in various primary immunodeficiencies, the reader is directed to **Table 1** for clinical correlations, and to **Fig. 1** for a mechanistic diagram.

DEFECTIVE TOLERANCE IN PRIMARY IMMUNODEFICIENCIES
Defects in Thymic Central Tolerance

Central tolerance refers to the deletion of autoreactive T cells during development in the thymus. Single positive thymocytes binding with overly high avidity to self-peptide-major histocompatibility complex undergo apoptosis in the thymic medulla, preventing escape of self-reactive T cells to the periphery (reviewed in[2]). This process relies in part on ectopic expression and presentation of proteins usually restricted to peripheral tissues, by medullary thymic epithelial cells (mTEC). Promiscuous expression of tissue-restricted antigens (TRAs) by mTEC is regulated by a transcription factor called the autoimmune regulator, or AIRE.[3] The mechanism through which AIRE activates expression of TRAs is not fully elucidated, but requires oligomerization, nuclear localization, DNA binding, and interactions with other nuclear factors,[4] and mutations affecting these functions cause autoimmune polyendocrinopathy, candidiasis, and ectodermal dysplasia (APECED), also known as autoimmune polyendocrinopathy syndrome type 1 (APS-1),[5,6] a disease characterized by multiorgan autoimmunity with loss of tolerance to AIRE-regulated gene products. The most common organs involved are parathyroid and adrenal glands, β cells in the islets of Langerhans, and the liver. Autoantibody formation against cytokines such as interleukin (IL)-17 and IL-22 may contribute to the immunodeficiency, increasing susceptibility to mucocutaneous candidal infection.[3,7] In addition, lack of expression of TRAs may lead to a failure in development of regulatory T cells (Treg),[8] causing impaired peripheral tolerance.

In animal models, AIRE expression in the thymus was shown to require cross-talk between developing thymocytes and stromal cells.[9] AIRE gene expression was shown to be decreased in the thymi of RAG-deficient patients with T-B-SCID and Omenn syndrome, in conjunction with lymphoid depletion and loss of corticomedullary differentiation.[10] A lack of expression of TRAs was observed, which may permit the few T-cell clones that develop to escape negative selection. The inflammatory manifestations of Omenn syndrome include T-cell-mediated inflammation in skin and intestine. Intestinal goblet cell and hair follicle antigens were shown in a murine model to be among the TRAs regulated by AIRE.[3]

Abnormal thymic development in DiGeorge syndrome (DGS) may result in impaired expression of AIRE, which may contribute to the autoimmunity seen in DGS.[11] Ten to 15% of patients with DGS have autoimmune disease,[12,13] most commonly idiopathic thrombocytopenic purpura, hemolytic anemia, thyroid disease, and juvenile idiopathic arthritis. The pathophysiology is thought to be a multifactorial failure of T-cell development with autoreactive T-cell escape and restricted Treg diversity.[14]

Central deletion can also be evaded due to abnormalities in TCR signaling, leading to defective activation-induced cell death (AICD). Null mutations in ZAP 70, a critical kinase downstream of the TCR, lead to combined immunodeficiency, by impairing positive selection in the thymus. In murine models, hypomorphic mutations in ZAP70 cause a syndrome of autoimmunity because of ineffective negative selection and reduced FoxP3+ Treg formation.[15] A human counterpart to this ZAP70-mediated autoimmune syndrome has not been identified. The store operated calcium entry (SOCE)-nuclear factor of activated T cells (NFAT) pathway is another signaling mechanism through which AICD is induced via the TCR. ORAI1, a calcium

Table 1
Correlation of genetic defects, mechanisms of impaired tolerance, and clinical autoimmune and inflammatory conditions in primary immunodeficiencies

Primary Immunodeficiency	Genetic Defect	Mechanisms	Autoimmune Features	Ref.
APECED	AIRE	• Impaired TRA presentation by mTECs • Impaired negative selection in thymic medulla • Impaired Treg development	• Hypoparathyroidism, hypothyroidism, adrenal insufficiency, type 1 diabetes, gonadal dysfunction, AIH, pernicious anemia, vitiligo, alopecia, primary biliary cirrhosis • Chronic mucocutaneous candidiasis	5–7,9,138
Omenn syndrome	Hypomorphic RAG1, RAG2, others	• Paucity of thymocytes • Defective thymic stromal, epithelial development • Decreased AIRE gene expression	• Destructive T-cell mediated inflammation in skin (erythroderma) and intestines • Lymphadenopathy, hepatosplenomegaly	10
ORAI1 deficiency	ORAI1	• Defective TCR mediated calcium flux and NFAT signaling • Defective AICD • Reduction of Tregs	• ITP, AIHA, lymphoproliferation	16,17
STIM1 deficiency	STIM1	• Defective TCR-mediated calcium flux and NFAT signaling • Reduction of Tregs	• ITP, AIHA, lymphoproliferation	18,19
DGS	Chromosome 22q11 deletion, TBX1	• Impaired thymic development and AIRE gene expression • Reduction in Treg numbers and function	• Hypoparathyroidism, ITP, AIHA, thyroid disease, and JRA	12–14,139,140
IPEX	FOXP3	• Impaired Treg development	• Severe early-onset enteropathy, type 1 diabetes, autoimmune cytopenias, hypothyroidism, eczema	44,45
IPEX-like	STAT5b, CD25, ITCH	• Impaired IL-2 receptor signaling • Impaired function, regulatory cytokine production by Treg • Dysregulated FoxP3 transcription	• Lymphoproliferation, IPEX-like autoimmunity	48–51

(continued on next page)

Table 1
(continued)

Primary Immunodeficiency	Genetic Defect	Mechanisms	Autoimmune Features	Ref.
CTLA-4 deficiency	CTLA-4	• Defective Treg development and function	• Enteropathy, GLILD, autoimmune cytopenias, hepatitis, thyroiditis, arthritis, psoriasis	53,54
LRBA deficiency	LRBA	• Impaired Treg survival	• Lymphoid interstitial pneumonia/GLILD, enteropathy, autoimmune cytopenias, thyroiditis, myasthenia gravis, atrophic gastritis	57–60
ALPS	FAS FAS ligand Caspase 8 Caspase 10 FADD PKC-δ	• Impaired FAS-mediated apoptosis	• Autoimmune cytopenias • Organ-specific autoimmunity • Lymphadenopathy, hepatosplenomegaly	23–27,36
	NRAS, KRAS	• Impaired mitochondrial apoptosis		29–31
Complement deficiencies	C1q, C1r, C1s, C4, C2	• Defective clearance of apoptotic bodies • Impaired clearance of immune complexes	• SLE, ANCA vasculitis	34,35
Hyper-IgM syndromes	CD40L/CD40	• Defective peripheral tolerance • Reduced Treg, elevated BAFF levels	• AIHA, chronic neutropenia, ITP, polyarthritis, IBD, biliary tract/liver disease, thyroiditis	82,141
	AID	• Defective central tolerance • Defective peripheral tolerance • Reduced Treg, elevated BAFF	• AIHA, ITP, polyarthritis, IBD, type I DM, AIH, chronic uveitis, lymphadenopathy	78–80
	UNG	• Unclear	• Lymphadenopathy	142
	NEMO IkBα	• Unclear	• Enteropathy, autoimmune cytopenias	143,144
XLA	BTK	• Impaired BCR signaling • Impaired central tolerance	• (Rare): JRA, RA, IBD, cytopenias, hypothyroidism, vasculitis, dermatomyositis	70,145

Disease	Genes	Mechanisms	Clinical features	References
CVID	Unknown in majority; TACI, ICOS, BAFF-R, CD19, CD20, CD21, CD81, MSH5	• Mechanisms unclear • Defective central tolerance in some (TACI mutations) • Reduced Treg • Elevated BAFF levels • Increased type 1 IFN signaling • Increased IL-12 in gut • IFN-γ in liver • TNF-αpolymorphisms • Defective BCR-mediated calcium signaling	• Autoimmune cytopenias • Enteropathy • GLILD • Hepatitis • Rheumatologic diseases	61–63,76,87,89, 106,108,116, 124,127
CGD	gp91phox, p22phox, p47phox, p67phox, p40phox	• Ineffective clearance of antigens leading to chronic stimulation, enhanced type 1 IFN signature • Defective induction of Tregs	• Colitis, discoid lupus, carriers with rheumatologic disease	38,39,41
Familial HLH	PRF1, UNC13D, STX11, STXBP2, RAB27A, LYST, AP3B	• Impaired cytotoxic function in • Persistence of DCs presenting viral antigen • Production of IFN-γ, IL-6, and TNF-α • Infiltration of tissues, bone marrow by hyperactivated, destructive histiocytes	• Severe inflammatory syndrome • Persistent fever • Hepatosplenomegaly • Liver dysfunction • Cytopenias • CNS inflammation	94–97
XLP	SH2D1A, XIAP	• Partially defective NK cell and CTL cytotoxic activity	• Lymphoproliferation • HLH	98
WAS	WASp	• Intrinsic signaling abnormality in B cells • Reduction in Treg numbers and function	• Thrombocytopenia, AIHA, neutropenia, IBD, arthritis, vasculitis, renal disease	65,146
Hyper-IgE syndrome	STAT3, DOCK8	• Altered Treg and cytokine signaling • Decreased number and function of Tregs • Autoreactive B cells	• Cytopenias, organ-specific autoimmunity (lung, gastrointestinal, hepatic, and/or endocrine), enteropathy, type 1 diabetes mellitus, lymphadenopathy • SLE	66,67

Abbreviations: AIHA, autoimmune hemolytic anemia; CNS, central nervous system; DM, diabetes mellitus; ITP, immune thrombocytopenia; JRA, juvenile rheumatoid arthritis; WAS, Wiskott-Aldrich syndrome; XLP, x-linked lymphoproliferative disease.
Data from Refs.[5–7,9,10,12–14,16–19,23–27,29–31,34–36,38,39,41,44,45,48–51,53,54,57–63,65–67,70,76,78–80,82,87,89,94–98,106,108,116,124,127,138–146]

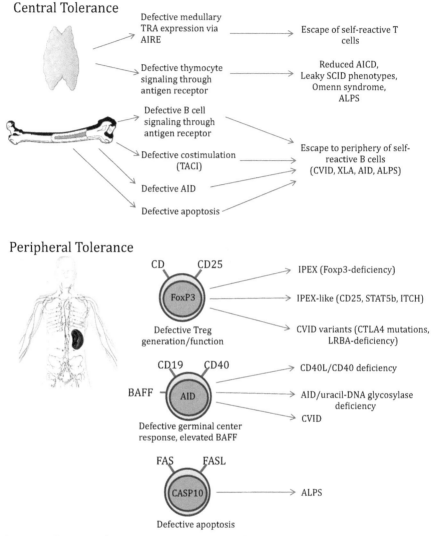

Fig. 1. Mechanisms of autoimmunity in PID disorders and some of the major mechanisms through which loss of self-tolerance and autoimmunity occur in PID syndromes, as discussed in the text.

release activated channel (CRAC channel), is a major route of calcium entry after TCR engagement, and its absence prevents apoptosis through reduced nuclear localization of NFAT.[16] ORAI1-deficiency in humans leads to severe combined immunodeficiency (SCID) with associated autoimmunity.[17] Deficiency in STIM1, an endoplasmic reticulum membrane protein responsible for activating CRAC channels during SOCE signaling, also presents with the combination of immunodeficiency and autoimmunity, arguing for defects in negative selection, although this relates at least in part to defects in Treg development and impaired peripheral tolerance.[18,19] Defective signaling leading to escape from AICD-mediated clonal deletion could conceivably explain the inflammatory diseases seen in other forms of hypomorphic or "leaky" SCID in humans. Additional defects in apoptosis and clonal deletion are discussed in the next section.

Apoptosis in Tolerance

Programmed cell death or apoptosis plays a key role in the elimination of self-reactive T and B cells at central and peripheral tolerance checkpoints.[20] Its importance in negative selection of lymphocytes was demonstrated with the discovery of a mutation in FAS, a member of the tumor necrosis factor (TNF) receptor family, in the autoimmune-prone MRL/lpr mouse.[21] FAS signals through a death-inducing signaling complex or DISC, which includes FAS-associated protein death domain (FADD) and caspase 8, to activate downstream caspases and ultimately apoptosis (reviewed in[22]).

The human homologue in which ineffective apoptosis leads to autoimmunity is autoimmune lymphoproliferative syndrome (ALPS). Patients present with lymphoproliferation, autoimmune cytopenias, and organ-specific autoimmunity (reviewed in[23]). The most common mutations in human ALPS affect FAS, involving either germline or somatic mutations. Mutations in Fas ligand,[24] caspase 10,[25] caspase 8,[26] FADD,[27] and protein kinase c δ (PKC-δ)[28] cause ALPS due to impaired FAS-mediated apoptosis. Furthermore, newer genetic causes of a phenotypically similar disease called RAS-associated autoimmune leukoproliferative disorder impair non-FAS-mediated mitochondrial apoptosis and include germline and somatic mutations in small GTPAses NRAS and KRAS.[29–31]

Defects in clearance of apoptotic bodies and immune complexes can lead to a breakdown in tolerance.[32] The classical complement pathway is required for safe elimination of immune complexes and apoptotic bodies.[33–35] Systemic lupus erythematosus (SLE) is found in association with classical complement deficiencies. SLE is found in 90% of patients with C1q deficiency, 75% of patients with complete C4 deficiency, 50% to 65% of patients with C1r/s deficiencies, and 10% to 30% of patients with C2 deficiency.[36,37] Homozygous C2 deficiency is the most common complement component deficiency.[36]

Defects in phagocyte function such as in chronic granulomatous disease (CGD) are also associated with autoimmune and inflammatory disease (reviewed in[38]). Functional oxidative burst in phagocytes is important in clearance of apoptotic cells and antigen, and defects in CGD are postulated to lead to prolonged inflammatory cell recruitment and cytokine production.[38] Notably, a prominent type I interferon (IFN) responsive gene expression signature was noted in murine models and humans with CGD mutations, in association with autoimmunity.[39] A similar gene expression profile has been shown in SLE, rheumatoid arthritis (RA), and Sjogren syndrome.[40] Furthermore, nicotinamide adenine dinucleotide phosphate (NAPDH) oxidase activity in macrophages is important for the induction of Tregs.[41]

Regulatory T Cells and Peripheral Tolerance

The critical role of a subset of CD4+ CD25+ T cells in maintaining peripheral tolerance was first demonstrated by Sakaguchi and colleagues[42] in murine models. Forkhead box protein P3 (Foxp3) is the central transcriptional regulator of the development and function of Treg.[43] Mutations in FOXP3 cause reductions in number and diversity of Tregs, and a severe break in peripheral tolerance leading to immune dysregulation, polyendocrinopathy, enteropathy, X-linked (IPEX), which is a profound autoimmune and inflammatory syndrome characterized clinically by intractable diarrhea, multiorgan autoimmunity, and eczema before 1 year of age.[44–46] Tregs depend on IL-2 signaling for development and function, and defects in IL-2 signaling lead to IPEX-like syndrome, with similar autoimmune and inflammatory manifestations.[47] These manifestations include mutations in the α chain of the IL-2 receptor (CD25),[48] and mutations in STAT5b, an intracellular mediator of IL-2 signaling.[49] Mutations in ITCH, which regulates FoxP3 transcription, also cause IPEX-like disease.[50,51] As discussed earlier, STIM1 deficiency in humans leads to reduced Tregs in the periphery, arguing for important roles for SOCE and NFAT signaling in their development.[18]

Other mutations found to cause defective Treg development and function, associated with autoimmune and lymphoproliferative disease in humans, include those in cytotoxic T-lymphocyte-associated protein 4 (CTLA-4) and lipopolysaccharide responsive beige-like anchor protein (LRBA). CTLA-4 is an inhibitory receptor constitutively expressed on Tregs, and upregulated on activated effector T cells (reviewed in[52]). CTLA-4 knockout mice display a severe autoimmune syndrome similar to IPEX.[53,54] Heterozygous CTLA-4 mutations were recently shown to cause a syndrome of immunodeficiency, autoimmunity, and lymphoproliferation in humans, with reduced Treg function.[55,56] This is particularly interesting from 2 perspectives. First, CTLA-4 heterozygous mice do not display an abnormal phenotype,[53] and second, the penetrance of the disease phenotype in humans is incomplete.[55,56] Treg function, however, is impaired in both healthy and affected family members with CTLA-4 mutations,[55] suggesting that although CTLA-4 haploinsufficiency affects Treg function in humans, other genetic or environmental factors may be required for manifestation of immunodeficiency, autoimmunity, and lymphoproliferation in this setting.

LRBA has been implicated in endosomal trafficking and cell survival, and its deficiency has been shown to have a selective effect on Treg survival, postulated to relate to impaired autophagy and abnormal mTOR signaling.[57,58] Homozygous LRBA deficiency in humans has recently been shown to impair Treg function and lead to a similar syndrome of immunodeficiency, autoimmunity, and lymphoproliferation.[57–60] Reductions in Treg numbers and function have been shown in other primary immunodeficiencies in which autoimmunity occurs, such as common variable immunodeficiency (CVID),[61–64] Wiskott-Aldrich syndrome,[65] hyper-immunoglobulin E (IgE) syndromes,[66,67] CGD,[41] and DGS.[68]

Central and Peripheral B-Cell Tolerance

The initial stages of B-cell development occur in the bone marrow, during which lymphoid progenitor cells progress through pro-B, pre-B, and immature B-cell stages and rearrange the B-cell receptor (BCR). The second stage occurs in lymphoid tissues, when B cells enter follicles, undergo class-switch recombination (CSR) and somatic hypermutation (SHM), and differentiate into memory B cells and antibody secreting plasma cells. The initial checkpoint to prevent emergence of self-reactive B cells from the bone marrow requires signaling through the newly rearranged BCR (reviewed in[69]). High signal strength results in receptor internalization and downregulation of the B-cell activating factor (BAFF) receptor, which reduces survival signaling to the developing B cell. In addition, high signal strength induces RAG gene activity, and subsequent receptor editing, allowing the cell another opportunity to rearrange a non-self-reactive receptor. If a less self-reactive receptor is not expressed within 1 to 2 days, the cell dies because of activation of the mitochondrial apoptosis pathway, which is unopposed due to downregulation of BAFF-R.

BCR signaling through Bruton tyrosine kinase (BTK) has been shown to play a role in central B-cell tolerance. Although few B cells develop in x-linked agammaglobulinemia (XLA) patients, those new emigrant/transitional B cells that emerge are enriched in self-reactive clones.[70] Antibody-mediated autoimmunity is rare in these patients however, because defective BCR signaling impairs antibody secretion in the periphery, and peripheral tolerance mechanisms are intact. Another signaling protein downstream of the BCR, PTPN22, has recently been recognized as important in tolerance, and polymorphisms in this gene are strongly associated with autoimmunity in patients with CVID and other primary antibody deficiencies.[71]

Toll-like receptor signaling was shown to be important in central B-cell tolerance, as patients with null mutations in IRAK-4 or MyD88 were shown to have a high frequency of self-reactive new emigrant/transitional B cells in circulation. However, autoantibody was not detected, and no clinical autoimmunity was reported, arguing that peripheral tolerance mechanisms are sufficient to prevent clinical manifestation of autoimmunity in these patients.[72]

Transmembrane activator, calcium modulator, and cyclophilin ligand interactor (TACI) mutations, occurring in 8% to 10% of patients with CVID,[73,74] are shown to increase susceptibility to autoimmunity and inflammation in those patients (reviewed in[75]). Individuals with mutations in TACI were shown to have a high frequency of self-reactive new emigrant/transitional B-cell clones escaping the bone marrow, which occurred in both CVID patients and healthy family members with heterozygous TACI mutations.[76] Interestingly, both TACI-mutant and non-TACI mutant CVID patients had self-reactive clones in the mature naïve B-cell compartment in the periphery, while healthy controls (whether TACI mutant or non-TACI mutant) did not. Thus, defective central tolerance due to TACI mutations was insufficient to cause autoimmunity, but in CVID patients, peripheral tolerance mechanisms were also defective, independent of TACI mutations. TACI mutations may therefore be disease modifiers in CVID, increasing the likelihood of autoimmunity by increasing the frequency of self-reactive clones escaping the bone marrow, but requiring additional lesions in peripheral tolerance for full manifestation of autoimmunity.

Activation-induced cytidine deaminase (AID) plays an important role in CSR and SHM. AID activity ultimately results in single-stranded DNA breaks, which are processed and repaired, allowing completion of CSR and SHM.[77] AID deficiency causes autosomal-recessive hyper-IgM syndrome, manifest by recurrent infections, lymphoid hyperplasia, and diverse autoimmune manifestations.[78,79] Although previously thought to be expressed only in germinal center B cells in the periphery, AID was recently shown to be expressed in immature B cells and play roles in both central and peripheral tolerance.[80] Impaired peripheral tolerance in AID patients correlated with increased circulating BAFF levels as well as reduced Treg frequency, the mechanisms for which were unclear.

Mutations in CD40-ligand (CD40L) affect peripheral tolerance. CD40/CD40L signaling plays roles in peripheral B-cell maturation, CSR, and SHM, as well as in optimal function of antigen-presenting/phagocytic cells and CTL. CD40L-deficient patients develop recurrent bacterial and opportunistic infections and frequent hematologic and organ-specific autoimmunity (reviewed in[81]). New emigrant/transitional B cells from CD40L-deficient patients were not enriched in self-reactive clones, suggesting that central B-cell tolerance was intact.[82] However, a higher proportion of autoreactive clones was found in the mature naïve B-cell compartment, arguing for defective peripheral tolerance. As in patients with AID deficiency, this correlated with elevated BAFF levels and reduced Treg, the latter presumed to be related to the previously demonstrated role of CD40-CD40L interactions in Treg development.[83]

Overexpression of BAFF in mice leads to B-cell hyperplasia, hypergammaglobulinemia, splenomegaly, and autoimmunity,[84] and is shown to rescue self-reactive B cells from deletion in the periphery, as well as facilitating entry into B-cell follicles.[85,86] Elevated serum BAFF levels have been found in patients with AID deficiency and CD40L deficiency (discussed earlier) as well as in patients with CVID and systemic autoimmune disease.[87,88] The mechanisms leading to its overexpression in these diseases are unclear.

Impaired calcium mobilization after BCR signaling has been shown in CVID patients prone to autoimmunity, granulomata, and splenomegaly.[89] Impaired BCR-induced calcium mobilization in these patients is associated with the expansion of CD21low B cells, a polyclonal population containing mostly autoreactive clones, expressing a gene profile suggestive of anergy, and a pattern of inflammatory chemokine receptors directing these cells to inflamed tissues.[90,91] The specific role these CD21low B cells play in autoimmune and inflammatory disease is unknown, but notably, similar CD21low B cell populations are seen in systemic lupus and RA patients.[90–92]

Contraction of the Immune Response

Hemophagocytic lymphohistiocytosis (HLH) is an inflammatory syndrome caused by impaired regulation of the adaptive immune response. Familial HLH is caused by mutations in genes, including UNC13D, STX11, STXBP2, RAB27A, LYST, and AP3B, involved in cytotoxic granule formation, trafficking or release, or encoding granule contents themselves (PRF1) (reviewed in[93]). Mice with mutations in these genes, which develop HLH in the setting of viral infection, have been helpful in understanding the mechanisms of HLH. Cytotoxic CD8+ T cells were found to regulate the number of dendritic cells (DCs) presenting viral antigen, such that in the setting of mutations affecting cytotoxicity, a larger number of DCs persisted and presented viral antigen.[94] Comparison of mice deficient in PRF1, LYST, RAB27A, STX11, and AP3B showed that the severity and timing of disease correlated with the degree of impairment in cytotoxicity and persistence of viral antigen, and a similar severity gradient was demonstrated in human disease caused by these various mutations.[95] The end result of this persistent antigen presentation is exuberant production of cytokines, including IFN-γ, IL-6, and TNF-α,[96] and a destructive infiltrative process with hyperactivated macrophages and histiocytes.[97] As discussed earlier, impaired antigen clearance causes abnormal cytokine expression and inflammatory disease in other settings, such as CGD. Other genetic defects causing HLH include SH2D1A, BIRC4, ITK, CD27, and MAGT1, which encode signaling proteins involved in activation of cytotoxic function as well as survival, differentiation, and migration of T and natural killer (NK) cells. Abnormalities in these genes result in susceptibility to HLH and lymphoproliferative disease (reviewed in[98]).

AUTOIMMUNE AND INFLAMMATORY COMPLICATIONS OF COMMON VARIABLE IMMUNODEFICIENCY

CVID is the most common clinically relevant PID, with prevalence estimated at 1:25,000. Although many single gene mutations are shown to present with a CVID phenotype (see **Table 1**), in most cases, no genetic lesion is known, and familial inheritance of CVID is rare.[99] CVID is frequently complicated by a wide range of autoimmune and inflammatory conditions, including enteropathy, granulomatous lymphocytic interstitial lung disease (GLILD), and liver disease, as well as lymphomas, which significantly shorten survival.[100–102] Abbott and colleagues,[147] have discussed the clinical aspects and management of these conditions in CVID patients. The mechanisms through which the autoimmune and inflammatory complications of CVID develop are not clear, but there has been a great deal of work on this in recent years, which is summarized in later discussion. Proposed mechanisms include many of those described earlier in monogenic primary immunodeficiencies. Furthermore, the diversity of mechanistic findings for each of these autoimmune and inflammatory complications highlights the likely polygenic and multifactorial nature of this disease.

Autoimmune Cytopenias and Rheumatologic Complications

Twenty percent of patients with CVID have associated autoimmunity.[99] Autoimmune cytopenias are the most common, and rheumatologic diseases, including a polyarticular arthritis resembling RA, occur in 10% to 30%.[103] This polyarthritis is distinct from RA in that it is typically seronegative, is nonerosive, and runs a benign course, resolving spontaneously.[104] Classic RA occurs less frequently, documented in 2% to 3% of CVID patients.[100,105]

A wide spectrum of additional systemic and organ-specific autoimmune diseases has been documented in CVID, including SLE, pernicious anemia, antiphospholipid syndrome, diabetes mellitus, juvenile RA, uveitis, multiple sclerosis, autoimmune thyroid disease, lichen planus, vasculitis, vitiligo, and psoriasis.[100,101]

Mechanistically, as discussed earlier, mutations in TACI may be found in 8% to 10% of CVID patients and seem to increase the predisposition to autoimmunity.[75] TACI mutations are shown to compromise central tolerance[76] and may thereby increase the risk of autoimmunity in these patients by increasing the frequency of self-reactive B cells escaping the bone marrow.

Peripheral tolerance was shown to be compromised in CVID patients regardless of TACI mutations,[76] and several potential lesions may contribute to this. The frequency and function of Treg cells are depressed in CVID patients with autoimmune cytopenias, thyroiditis, polyendocrinopathy, arthritis, and inflammatory manifestations including granulomatous disease and enteropathy.[61-63] Prosurvival signaling and entry of self-reactive cells into otherwise restricted B-cell follicles are allowed via elevated circulating BAFF levels in CVID patients.[87,106] Calcium signaling through the BCR is dysfunctional in a subgroup of CVID patients prone to autoimmunity and infiltrative disease[89]; correlating with poor class-switching and memory formation, and expansion of anergic, CD21lo B cells, with altered trafficking properties.[90-92] Interestingly, similar CD21lo populations have been shown in SLE and RA, and in fact, infiltrate synovial tissues.[90,91,107] The specific role of these cells is unclear. Last, an IFN-responsive gene expression signature is noted in CVID patients with autoimmunity, similar to SLE and RA patients.[40,108]

In summary, a plethora of potential mechanisms may explain the autoimmune and rheumatologic complications of CVID, including breakdown in central tolerance, and several defects affecting peripheral tolerance, expansion of abnormal B-cell populations with altered trafficking and effector functions, and altered cytokine expression and signaling.

Enteropathy

Noninfectious gastrointestinal disease occurs in 9% to 15% of CVID patients.[100,109] Histologically, findings in the small intestine include villous blunting, increased intraepithelial lymphocytes (IELs), mild duodenitis, and nodular lymphoid hyperplasia.[110,111] Findings in stomach include chronic gastritis, ranging from mild to severe mucosal atrophy in the body and antrum, with vitamin B12 deficiency and serologic evidence of pernicious anemia.[111,112] Graft versus host disease (GVHD)-like pathologic abnormality has been demonstrated in the colon.[111] Of note, a paucity of plasma cells in the gastrointestinal mucosa has been a unifying finding among these studies.[111,112]

The pathophysiology of CVID-enteropathy remains unclear. Parallels have been drawn with celiac disease, given the frequent findings of villous blunting and epithelial atrophy in a spruelike pattern. However, several studies have addressed the frequency of celiac-specific HLA haplotypes (HLA DQ2, DQ8) in CVID patients with enteropathy and have found no clear correlation, nor does the presence of these haplotypes in CVID patients portend responsiveness to gluten withdrawal.[111,113,114]

Regarding the absence of plasma cells in the gastrointestinal mucosa, gene expression analysis in the jejunum of B cell and IgA-deficient mice identified a "trialogue" between adaptive immunity, jejunal mucosal enterocytes, and intestinal microbiota.[115] When germ-free mice were populated by normal microbiota, gene expression in jejunal enterocytes was characterized by a Gata4-regulated metabolic pattern dictating fat absorption and leptin expression. In the absence of B cells or IgA, this switched to an IFN-responsive gene expression pattern. Similar IFN-response profiles were found in duodenal biopsies from CVID patients. This study suggests an interesting interplay between plasma cell-mediated mucosal IgA production, the intestinal microbiome, and enterocytes in setting the stage for intestinal inflammation in CVID.

Lamina propria mononuclear cells (LPMCs) isolated from intestinal biopsies from CVID patients with enteropathy produced significantly more IL-12 and IFN-γ, when stimulated in culture with innate stimuli or via the TCR, than LPMCs from CVID patients without enteropathy.[116] When compared with LPMCs from patients with Crohn disease, similar levels of IL-12 and IFN-γ were produced, but significantly less IL-23, IL-17, and TNF. Thus, CVID enteropathy involves a T-cell-mediated inflammatory process driven by IL-12 and IFN-γ, which is distinct from Crohn disease.

A role for impaired regulatory T-cell function in this condition is suspected given the recent findings of CTLA-4 mutations affecting Treg function, in patients who meet criteria for and were previously diagnosed with CVID,[55,56] as discussed earlier. Malabsorptive enteropathy was the most common clinical manifestation of immune dysregulation in those studies. The incomplete penetrance of this phenotype argues that heterozygous CTLA-4 mutations, which affect the function of Treg, may be disease modifiers in CVID, enhancing the susceptibility of CVID patients to autoimmune and inflammatory complications but requiring additional mutations or environmental factors to manifest clinically. Similarly, hypogammaglobulinemia, autoimmunity, and inflammatory enteropathy were shown in patients with homozygous mutations in LRBA, which are known to affect Treg survival and function,[57-60] and CTLA4 protein expression.[117]

Last, a genome-wide association study (GWAS) by Orange and colleagues[118] showed a strong association between CVID enteropathy and a polymorphism in the CACNA1C gene on chromosome 12; this is the αsubunit of a voltage-gated calcium channel, which has been shown to play a role in smooth muscle motility in rat intestine.[119] The specific role of this polymorphism in immunoregulation or the pathophysiology of CVID enteropathy has not yet been determined.

In summary, CVID is complicated by noninfectious enteropathy at a rate of 9% to 15%, and this subpopulation is at increased risk for autoimmune disease and death. Characteristic features include villous blunting, increased IELs, and nodular lymphoid hyperplasia in the small bowel, and GVHD-like apoptosis in the colon, with a paucity of plasma cells in the mucosa. The pathophysiology remains unclear, although it may involve changes in innate immune signaling by enterocytes due to reduced mucosal IgA, reduced Treg function, and an IL-12 and IFN-γ-driven T-cell-mediated inflammatory process.

Granulomatous Lymphocytic Infiltrative Lung Disease

Noninfectious lung disease in CVID includes bronchiectasis, isolated granulomata, and a more diffuse infiltrative process that involves loose granulomata and a mixed infiltrate of T cells, B cells, histiocytes, and stromal cells, which has recently been named granulomatous interstitial lung disease, or GLILD.[102]

The histopathology of GLILD has been studied in depth.[120] It has been described as an expansion of bronchus-associated lymphoid tissue (BALT), tertiary lymphoid neogenesis in the lung, or pulmonary lymphoid hyperplasia (PLH), and involves a variable lymphocytic infiltrative process with formation of ectopic germinal centers. PLH may present in several histologic patterns, including those of lymphocytic interstitial pneumonia, follicular bronchiolitis, nodular lymphoid hyperplasia, and reactive lymphoid hyperplasia. All of these include mixed infiltrates of T cells, B cells, antigen presenting cells, stromal cells, and loosely organized granulomata, all of which fall under the umbrella term GLILD. Peribronchial lymphocytic infiltrates in this process are organized into CD20+ B-cell-rich follicles surrounded by more diffuse T-cell zones. Follicles are Ki67 and Bcl6+ and contained CD23+ follicular DCs, identifying these as actively proliferating ectopic germinal centers. In general, there is a predominance of CD4+ T cells. Tertiary lymphoid neogenesis occurs in other autoimmune and inflammatory diseases, including Sjogren syndrome and RA. These diseases have been shown to be responsive to B-cell depletion therapies, arguing that these ectopic B-cell-rich germinal centers may drive the expansion or persistence of the infiltrative process.[120]

In murine models, the development of BALT is dependent on follicular dendritic cells, which in turn require lymphotoxin α/β (LT$\alpha\beta$) and CXCL13 (reviewed in[121]). In mice, depletion of dendritic cells or inhibition of lymphotoxin can induce regression of BALT. Treg have been shown to inhibit the formation of BALT in mice. Pulmonary disease is a rare manifestation of human IPEX,[122] but GLILD is seen frequently in patients with mutations in CTLA-4[55,56] and LRBA,[57,58] arguing that abnormalities of Treg function may contribute to this process.

TNF-α is known to play a key role in granuloma formation[123] and may play a role in granulomatous disease and GLILD in CVID patients. An uncommon TNF-α polymorphism was shown to correlate significantly with the occurrence of pulmonary granulomatous disease and splenomegaly in CVID.[124]

A role for chronic viral infection in GLILD pathogenesis was proposed, and one group has shown an association between PCR positivity for human herpesvirus 8 and GLILD, while others have not seen the same association.[125,126]

Last, a role for stromal cell function in the pathogenesis of GLILD is suggested by the finding of a single nucleotide polymorphism (SNP) in the FGF14 gene found to be highly associated with lymphoid interstitial pneumonitis in CVID patients in the GWAS study mentioned previously.[118]

In summary, GLILD is an infiltrative disease of the lung, involving tertiary lymphoid neogenesis. The pathogenesis is not well understood, but murine studies have demonstrated roles for LT$\alpha\beta$ and follicular DCs in tertiary lymphoid neogenesis and formation of BALT, and Treg in regulating its formation. Treg dysfunction may predispose to GLILD in CVID, as evidenced by the prevalence of GLILD in the setting of mutations in CTLA-4 or LRBA, which have clear impacts on Treg function. TNF-α polymorphisms may play a role in granulomatous disease in CVID. Chronic viral infection could be a trigger or driver in the formation of GLILD in CVID patients, although this is in debate. The strong association of GLILD with a polymorphism in FGF14 suggests an as-yet unexplored role of stromal cells in this inflammatory disease.

Nodular Regenerative Hyperplasia and Autoimmune Hepatitis

Noninfectious liver disease occurs in 5% to 12% of CVID patients[127,128] and shortens survival.[100] Most CVID patients biopsied to evaluate hepatic disease had nodular regenerative hyperplasia (NRH), characterized by diffuse transformation of the hepatic parenchyma into small, regenerative nodules, without significant fibrosis.[129,130] In CVID, intrasinusoidal lymphocytic infiltrates of CD8+ T cells are often present in conjunction with this.[127,130] Importantly, portal hypertension, a known complication of NRH, was present in 20% to 75%.[127,128,130]

In a subsequent study, more than half of the patients had associated portal and lobular inflammatory infiltrates, sometimes occurring in conjunction with interface hepatitis and bridging necrosis, which was termed autoimmune hepatitis (AIH)-like disease. Of note, there was a paucity of plasma cells in biopsies. Interestingly, in one patient, followed with serial biopsies over 6 years, the disease was shown to progress from mild NRH to this more severe AIH-like illness. The interface hepatitis in these patients was shown to involve CD8+ T cells and IFN-γ expression. Furthermore, patients with this AIH-like disease, unlike typical NRH, developed hepatic synthetic dysfunction in addition to portal HTN.

NRH occurs in other disease settings as well, including autoimmune and hematologic illnesses and infections, and in the setting of treatment with certain medications (reviewed in[129]). The prevalence of NRH in autopsy studies is approximately 2%.[131,132] Interestingly, the frequency with which portal hypertension is found in association with NRH in autopsy studies was low, at 4.7%,[131] arguing that both the frequency and the severity of this entity may be increased in CVID patients.

The underlying cause of NRH is thought to involve disturbances in perfusion in the hepatic microvasculature, leading to a local hyperplastic response in hepatocytes,[129] possibly caused by congenital anomalies in portal vasculature, hematologic or prothrombotic disorders, toxic, or immunologic injury to endothelial cells.[129,133,134] CD8+ T cells may play a role in pathogenesis in some patients.[134] Cytokines, including IFN-γ[127] and IL-6,[135] have been postulated to play roles in this disease. Autoantibodies, particularly antiphospholipid antibodies contributing to prothrombotic states, have been shown in association with NRH and may play a role in some patients.[136] In the GWAS study cited earlier, NRH in CVID patients was significantly associated with 2 SNPs on chromosome 1, the specific identity and function of which are unknown.[118] Other polymorphisms or single-gene mutations mentioned in previous sections on enteropathy and GLILD, such as CTLA-4, LRBA, and TNF-α, have not been clearly associated with NRH. That being said, infiltrative liver disease and hepatomegaly were noted in patients with CTLA-4 mutations,[55] and hepatitis has been seen in a minority of patients with IPEX,[137] arguing that the more severe AIH-like variant discussed earlier may be related to abnormalities in T-cell regulation or Treg function.

SUMMARY

Identification of genetic lesions in primary immunodeficiencies complicated by autoimmune and inflammatory diseases has illuminated numerous mechanisms bridging immune development with central and peripheral tolerance, and regulation of the immune response. This knowledge is facilitating advancements in the understanding of more complex, multifactorial syndromes of autoimmunity and immunodeficiency, such as CVID, SLE, and RA, and it is hoped will soon lead to advancements in therapy for these diseases.

REFERENCES

1. Ozen S, Bilginer Y. A clinical guide to autoinflammatory diseases: familial Mediterranean fever and next-of-kin. Nat Rev Rheumatol 2014;10(3):135–47.
2. Klein L, Kyewski B, Allen PM, et al. Positive and negative selection of the T cell repertoire: what thymocytes see (and don't see). Nat Rev Immunol 2014;14(6):377–91.
3. Anderson MS, Venanzi ES, Klein L, et al. Projection of an immunological self shadow within the thymus by the AIRE protein. Science 2002;298(5597): 1395–401.

4. Zumer K, Saksela K, Peterlin BM. The mechanism of tissue-restricted antigen gene expression by AIRE. J Immunol 2013;190(6):2479–82.
5. Nagamine K, Peterson P, Scott HS, et al. Positional cloning of the APECED gene. Nat Genet 1997;17(4):393–8.
6. De Martino L, Capalbo D, Improda N, et al. APECED: a paradigm of complex interactions between genetic background and susceptibility factors. Front Immunol 2013;4:331.
7. Puel A, Doffinger R, Natividad A, et al. Autoantibodies against IL-17A, IL-17F, and IL-22 in patients with chronic mucocutaneous candidiasis and autoimmune polyendocrine syndrome type I. J Exp Med 2010;207(2):291–7.
8. Su MA, Anderson MS. AIRE: an update. Curr Opin Immunol 2004;16(6):746–52.
9. Zuklys S, Balciunaite G, Agarwal A, et al. Normal thymic architecture and negative selection are associated with AIRE expression, the gene defective in the autoimmune-polyendocrinopathy-candidiasis-ectodermal dystrophy (APECED). J Immunol 2000;165(4):1976–83.
10. Cavadini P, Vermi W, Facchetti F, et al. AIRE deficiency in thymus of 2 patients with Omenn syndrome. J Clin Invest 2005;115(3):728–32.
11. Capalbo D, Giardino G, Martino LD, et al. Genetic basis of altered central tolerance and autoimmune diseases: a lesson from AIRE mutations. Int Rev Immunol 2012;31(5):344–62.
12. Jawad AF, McDonald-Mcginn DM, Zackai E, et al. Immunologic features of chromosome 22q11.2 deletion syndrome (DiGeorge syndrome/velocardiofacial syndrome). J Pediatr 2001;139(5):715–23.
13. Gennery AR, Barge D, O'Sullivan JJ, et al. Antibody deficiency and autoimmunity in 22q11.2 deletion syndrome. Arch Dis Child 2002;86(6):422–5.
14. Ferrando-Martinez S, Lorente R, Gurbindo D, et al. Low thymic output, peripheral homeostasis deregulation, and hastened regulatory T cells differentiation in children with 22q11.2 deletion syndrome. J Pediatr 2014;164(4):882–9.
15. Siggs OM, Miosge LA, Yates AL, et al. Opposing functions of the T cell receptor kinase ZAP-70 in immunity and tolerance differentially titrate in response to nucleotide substitutions. Immunity 2007;27(6):912–26.
16. Kim KD, Srikanth S, Yee MK, et al. ORAI1 deficiency impairs activated T cell death and enhances T cell survival. J Immunol 2011;187(7):3620–30.
17. McCarl CA, Picard C, Khalil S, et al. ORAI1 deficiency and lack of store-operated Ca2+ entry cause immunodeficiency, myopathy, and ectodermal dysplasia. J Allergy Clin Immunol 2009;124(6):1311–8.e17.
18. Picard C, McCarl CA, Papolos A, et al. STIM1 mutation associated with a syndrome of immunodeficiency and autoimmunity. N Engl J Med 2009;360(19):1971–80.
19. Oh-Hora M, Yamashita M, Hogan PG, et al. Dual functions for the endoplasmic reticulum calcium sensors STIM1 and STIM2 in T cell activation and tolerance. Nat Immunol 2008;9(4):432–43.
20. Lenardo M, Chan KM, Hornung F, et al. Mature T lymphocyte apoptosis–immune regulation in a dynamic and unpredictable antigenic environment. Annu Rev Immunol 1999;17:221–53.
21. Watanabe-Fukunaga R, Brannan CI, Copeland NG, et al. Lymphoproliferation disorder in mice explained by defects in Fas antigen that mediates apoptosis. Nature 1992;356(6367):314–7.
22. Wilson NS, Dixit V, Ashkenazi A. Death receptor signal transducers: nodes of coordination in immune signaling networks. Nat Immunol 2009;10(4):348–55.
23. Oliveira JB. The expanding spectrum of the autoimmune lymphoproliferative syndromes. Curr Opin Pediatr 2013;25(6):722–9.

24. Del-Rey M, Ruiz-Contreras J, Bosque A, et al. A homozygous Fas ligand gene mutation in a patient causes a new type of autoimmune lymphoproliferative syndrome. Blood 2006;108(4):1306–12.

25. Wang J, Zheng L, Lobito A, et al. Inherited human Caspase 10 mutations underlie defective lymphocyte and dendritic cell apoptosis in autoimmune lymphoproliferative syndrome type II. Cell 1999;98(1):47–58.

26. Chun HJ, Zheng L, Ahmad M, et al. Pleiotropic defects in lymphocyte activation caused by caspase-8 mutations lead to human immunodeficiency. Nature 2002; 419(6905):395–9.

27. Bolze A, Byun M, McDonald D, et al. Whole-exome-sequencing-based discovery of human FADD deficiency. Am J Hum Genet 2010;87(6):873–81.

28. Kuehn HS, Niemela JE, Rangel-Santos A, et al. Loss-of-function of the protein kinase C delta (PKCdelta) causes a B-cell lymphoproliferative syndrome in humans. Blood 2013;121(16):3117–25.

29. Oliveira JB, Bidere N, Niemela JE, et al. NRAS mutation causes a human autoimmune lymphoproliferative syndrome. Proc Natl Acad Sci U S A 2007;104(21): 8953–8.

30. Niemela JE, Lu L, Fleisher TA, et al. Somatic KRAS mutations associated with a human nonmalignant syndrome of autoimmunity and abnormal leukocyte homeostasis. Blood 2011;117(10):2883–6.

31. Takagi M, Shinoda K, Piao J, et al. Autoimmune lymphoproliferative syndrome-like disease with somatic KRAS mutation. Blood 2011;117(10):2887–90.

32. Arason GJ, Jorgensen GH, Ludviksson BR. Primary immunodeficiency and autoimmunity: lessons from human diseases. Scand J Immunol 2010;71(5):317–28.

33. Pickering MC, Botto M, Taylor PR, et al. Systemic lupus erythematosus, complement deficiency, and apoptosis. Adv Immunol 2000;76:227–324.

34. Arason GJ, Geirsson AJ, Kolka R, et al. Deficiency of complement-dependent prevention of immune precipitation in systemic sclerosis. Ann Rheum Dis 2002;61(3):257–60.

35. Arason GJ, Steinsson K, Kolka R, et al. Patients with systemic lupus erythematosus are deficient in complement-dependent prevention of immune precipitation. Rheumatology 2004;43(6):783–9.

36. Bussone G, Mouthon L. Autoimmune manifestations in primary immune deficiencies. Autoimmun Rev 2009;8(4):332–6.

37. Etzioni A. Immune deficiency and autoimmunity. Autoimmun Rev 2003;2(6): 364–9.

38. Kang EM, Marciano BE, DeRavin S, et al. Chronic granulomatous disease: overview and hematopoietic stem cell transplantation. J Allergy Clin Immunol 2011; 127(6):1319–26 [quiz: 1327–8].

39. Kelkka T, Kienhofer D, Hoffmann M, et al. Reactive oxygen species deficiency induces autoimmunity with type 1 interferon signature. Antioxid Redox Signal 2014;21(16):2231–45.

40. Toro-Dominguez D, Carmona-Saez P, Alarcon-Riquelme ME. Shared signatures between rheumatoid arthritis, systemic lupus erythematosus and Sjogren's syndrome uncovered through gene expression meta-analysis. Arthritis Res Ther 2014;16(6):489.

41. Kraaij MD, Savage ND, van der Kooij SW, et al. Induction of regulatory T cells by macrophages is dependent on production of reactive oxygen species. Proc Natl Acad Sci U S A 2010;107(41):17686–91.

42. Sakaguchi S, Sakaguchi N, Asano M, et al. Immunologic self-tolerance maintained by activated T cells expressing IL-2 receptor alpha-chains (CD25).

Breakdown of a single mechanism of self-tolerance causes various autoimmune diseases. J Immunol 1995;155(3):1151–64.

43. Fontenot JD, Gavin MA, Rudensky AY. Foxp3 programs the development and function of CD4+CD25+ regulatory T cells. Nat Immunol 2003;4(4):330–6.

44. Bennett CL, Christie J, Ramsdell F, et al. The immune dysregulation, polyendocrinopathy, enteropathy, X-linked syndrome (IPEX) is caused by mutations of FOXP3. Nat Genet 2001;27(1):20–1.

45. Wildin RS, Ramsdell F, Peake J, et al. X-linked neonatal diabetes mellitus, enteropathy and endocrinopathy syndrome is the human equivalent of mouse scurfy. Nat Genet 2001;27(1):18–20.

46. Chatila TA, Blaeser F, Ho N, et al. JM2, encoding a fork head-related protein, is mutated in X-linked autoimmunity-allergic dysregulation syndrome. J Clin Invest 2000;106(12):R75–81.

47. Zhang L, Zhao Y. The regulation of Foxp3 expression in regulatory CD4(+) CD25(+)T cells: multiple pathways on the road. J Cell Physiol 2007;211(3): 590–7.

48. Caudy AA, Reddy ST, Chatila T, et al. CD25 deficiency causes an immune dysregulation, polyendocrinopathy, enteropathy, X-linked-like syndrome, and defective IL-10 expression from CD4 lymphocytes. J Allergy Clin Immunol 2007;119(2):482–7.

49. Cohen AC, Nadeau KC, Tu W, et al. Cutting edge: decreased accumulation and regulatory function of CD4+ CD25(high) T cells in human STAT5b deficiency. J Immunol 2006;177(5):2770–4.

50. Lohr NJ, Molleston JP, Strauss KA, et al. Human ITCH E3 ubiquitin ligase deficiency causes syndromic multisystem autoimmune disease. Am J Hum Genet 2010;86(3):447–53.

51. Venuprasad K, Huang H, Harada Y, et al. The E3 ubiquitin ligase Itch regulates expression of transcription factor Foxp3 and airway inflammation by enhancing the function of transcription factor TIEG1. Nat Immunol 2008;9(3):245–53.

52. Sansom DM, Walker LS. The role of CD28 and cytotoxic T-lymphocyte antigen-4 (CTLA-4) in regulatory T-cell biology. Immunol Rev 2006;212:131–48.

53. Waterhouse P, Penninger JM, Timms E, et al. Lymphoproliferative disorders with early lethality in mice deficient in Ctla-4. Science 1995;270(5238):985–8.

54. Tivol EA, Borriello F, Schweitzer AN, et al. Loss of CTLA-4 leads to massive lymphoproliferation and fatal multiorgan tissue destruction, revealing a critical negative regulatory role of CTLA-4. Immunity 1995;3(5):541–7.

55. Schubert D, Bode C, Kenefeck R, et al. Autosomal dominant immune dysregulation syndrome in humans with CTLA4 mutations. Nat Med 2014;20(12): 1410–6.

56. Kuehn HS, Ouyang W, Lo B, et al. Immune dysregulation in human subjects with heterozygous germline mutations in CTLA4. Science 2014;345(6204):1623–7.

57. Charbonnier LM, Janssen E, Chou J, et al. Regulatory T-cell deficiency and immune dysregulation, polyendocrinopathy, enteropathy, X-linked-like disorder caused by loss-of-function mutations in LRBA. J Allergy Clin Immunol 2015; 135(1):217–27.e219.

58. Lopez-Herrera G, Tampella G, Pan-Hammarstrom Q, et al. Deleterious mutations in LRBA are associated with a syndrome of immune deficiency and autoimmunity. Am J Hum Genet 2012;90(6):986–1001.

59. Serwas NK, Kansu A, Santos-Valente E, et al. Atypical manifestation of LRBA deficiency with predominant IBD-like phenotype. Inflamm Bowel Dis 2015; 21(1):40–7.

60. Alangari A, Alsultan A, Adly N, et al. LPS-responsive beige-like anchor (LRBA) gene mutation in a family with inflammatory bowel disease and combined immunodeficiency. J Allergy Clin Immunol 2012;130(2):481–8.e2.

61. Fevang B, Yndestad A, Sandberg WJ, et al. Low numbers of regulatory T cells in common variable immunodeficiency: association with chronic inflammation in vivo. Clin Exp Immunol 2007;147(3):521–5.

62. Yu GP, Chiang D, Song SJ, et al. Regulatory T cell dysfunction in subjects with common variable immunodeficiency complicated by autoimmune disease. Clin Immunol 2009;131(2):240–53.

63. Arumugakani G, Wood PM, Carter CR. Frequency of Treg cells is reduced in CVID patients with autoimmunity and splenomegaly and is associated with expanded CD21lo B lymphocytes. J Clin Immunol 2010;30(2):292–300.

64. Genre J, Errante PR, Kokron CM, et al. Reduced frequency of CD4(+) CD25(HIGH)FOXP3(+) cells and diminished FOXP3 expression in patients with common variable immunodeficiency: a link to autoimmunity? Clin Immunol 2009;132(2):215–21.

65. Maillard MH, Cotta-de-Almeida V, Takeshima F, et al. The Wiskott-Aldrich syndrome protein is required for the function of CD4(+)CD25(+)Foxp3(+) regulatory T cells. J Exp Med 2007;204(2):381–91.

66. Milner JD, Vogel TP, Forbes L, et al. Early-onset lymphoproliferation and autoimmunity caused by germline STAT3 gain-of-function mutations. Blood 2015; 125(4):591–9.

67. Janssen E, Morbach H, Ullas S, et al. Dedicator of cytokinesis 8-deficient patients have a breakdown in peripheral B-cell tolerance and defective regulatory T cells. J Allergy Clin Immunol 2014;134(6):1365–74.

68. Sullivan KE, McDonald-McGinn D, Zackai EH. CD4(+) CD25(+) T-cell production in healthy humans and in patients with thymic hypoplasia. Clin Diagn Lab Immunol 2002;9(5):1129–31.

69. Goodnow CC, Sprent J, Fazekas de St Groth B, et al. Cellular and genetic mechanisms of self tolerance and autoimmunity. Nature 2005;435(7042):590–7.

70. Ng YS, Wardemann H, Chelnis J, et al. Bruton's tyrosine kinase is essential for human B cell tolerance. J Exp Med 2004;200(7):927–34.

71. Chew GY, Sinha U, Gatenby PA, et al. Autoimmunity in primary antibody deficiency is associated with protein tyrosine phosphatase nonreceptor type 22 (PTPN22). J Allergy Clin Immunol 2013;131(4):1130–5, 1135.e1.

72. Isnardi I, Ng YS, Srdanovic I, et al. IRAK-4- and MyD88-dependent pathways are essential for the removal of developing autoreactive B cells in humans. Immunity 2008;29(5):746–57.

73. Castigli E, Wilson SA, Garibyan L, et al. TACI is mutant in common variable immunodeficiency and IgA deficiency. Nat Genet 2005;37(8):829–34.

74. Salzer U, Chapel HM, Webster AD, et al. Mutations in TNFRSF13B encoding TACI are associated with common variable immunodeficiency in humans. Nat Genet 2005;37(8):820–8.

75. Lee JJ, Ozcan E, Rauter I, et al. Transmembrane activator and calcium-modulator and cyclophilin ligand interactor mutations in common variable immunodeficiency. Curr Opin Allergy Clin Immunol 2008;8(6):520–6.

76. Romberg N, Chamberlain N, Saadoun D, et al. CVID-associated TACI mutations affect autoreactive B cell selection and activation. J Clin Invest 2013;123(10): 4283–93.

77. Notarangelo LD, Lanzi G, Peron S, et al. Defects of class-switch recombination. J Allergy Clin Immunol 2006;117(4):855–64.

78. Quartier P, Bustamante J, Sanal O, et al. Clinical, immunologic and genetic analysis of 29 patients with autosomal recessive hyper-IgM syndrome due to Activation-Induced Cytidine Deaminase deficiency. Clin Immunol 2004;110(1): 22–9.
79. Revy P, Muto T, Levy Y, et al. Activation-induced cytidine deaminase (AID) deficiency causes the autosomal recessive form of the Hyper-IgM syndrome (HIGM2). Cell 2000;102(5):565–75.
80. Meyers G, Ng YS, Bannock JM, et al. Activation-induced cytidine deaminase (AID) is required for B-cell tolerance in humans. Proc Natl Acad Sci U S A 2011;108(28):11554–9.
81. Jesus AA, Duarte AJ, Oliveira JB. Autoimmunity in hyper-IgM syndrome. J Clin Immunol 2008;28(Suppl 1):S62–6.
82. Herve M, Isnardi I, Ng YS, et al. CD40 ligand and MHC class II expression are essential for human peripheral B cell tolerance. J Exp Med 2007;204(7): 1583–93.
83. Kumanogoh A, Wang X, Lee I, et al. Increased T cell autoreactivity in the absence of CD40-CD40 ligand interactions: a role of CD40 in regulatory T cell development. J Immunol 2001;166(1):353–60.
84. Stohl W, Xu D, Kim KS, et al. BAFF overexpression and accelerated glomerular disease in mice with an incomplete genetic predisposition to systemic lupus erythematosus. Arthritis Rheum 2005;52(7):2080–91.
85. Thien M, Phan TG, Gardam S, et al. Excess BAFF rescues self-reactive B cells from peripheral deletion and allows them to enter forbidden follicular and marginal zone niches. Immunity 2004;20(6):785–98.
86. Lesley R, Xu Y, Kalled SL, et al. Reduced competitiveness of autoantigen-engaged B cells due to increased dependence on BAFF. Immunity 2004; 20(4):441–53.
87. Knight AK, Radigan L, Marron T, et al. High serum levels of BAFF, APRIL, and TACI in common variable immunodeficiency. Clin Immunol 2007;124(2):182–9.
88. Mackay F, Sierro F, Grey ST, et al. The BAFF/APRIL system: an important player in systemic rheumatic diseases. Curr Dir Autoimmun 2005;8:243–65.
89. Foerster C, Voelxen N, Rakhmanov M, et al. B cell receptor-mediated calcium signaling is impaired in B lymphocytes of type Ia patients with common variable immunodeficiency. J Immunol 2010;184(12):7305–13.
90. Rakhmanov M, Keller B, Gutenberger S, et al. Circulating CD21low B cells in common variable immunodeficiency resemble tissue homing, innate-like B cells. Proc Natl Acad Sci U S A 2009;106(32):13451–6.
91. Isnardi I, Ng YS, Menard L, et al. Complement receptor 2/CD21- human naive B cells contain mostly autoreactive unresponsive clones. Blood 2010;115(24): 5026–36.
92. Wehr C, Kivioja T, Schmitt C, et al. The EUROclass trial: defining subgroups in common variable immunodeficiency. Blood 2008;111(1):77–85.
93. Chandrakasan S, Filipovich AH. Hemophagocytic lymphohistiocytosis: advances in pathophysiology, diagnosis, and treatment. J Pediatr 2013;163(5): 1253–9.
94. Terrell CE, Jordan MB. Perforin deficiency impairs a critical immunoregulatory loop involving murine CD8(+) T cells and dendritic cells. Blood 2013;121(26): 5184–91.
95. Jessen B, Kogl T, Sepulveda FE, et al. Graded defects in cytotoxicity determine severity of hemophagocytic lymphohistiocytosis in humans and mice. Front Immunol 2013;4:448.

96. Henter JI, Elinder G, Soder O, et al. Hypercytokinemia in familial hemophago-cytic lymphohistiocytosis. Blood 1991;78(11):2918–22.

97. Henter JI, Horne A, Arico M, et al. HLH-2004: diagnostic and therapeutic guide-lines for hemophagocytic lymphohistiocytosis. Pediatr Blood Cancer 2007; 48(2):124–31.

98. Parvaneh N, Filipovich AH, Borkhardt A. Primary immunodeficiencies predis-posed to Epstein-Barr virus-driven haematological diseases. Br J Haematol 2013;162(5):573–86.

99. Cunningham-Rundles C, Bodian C. Common variable immunodeficiency: clin-ical and immunological features of 248 patients. Clin Immunol 1999;92(1): 34–48.

100. Resnick ES, Moshier EL, Godbold JH, et al. Morbidity and mortality in common variable immune deficiency over 4 decades. Blood 2012;119(7):1650–7.

101. Chapel H, Lucas M, Lee M, et al. Common variable immunodeficiency disorders: division into distinct clinical phenotypes. Blood 2008;112(2): 277–86.

102. Bates CA, Ellison MC, Lynch DA, et al. Granulomatous-lymphocytic lung dis-ease shortens survival in common variable immunodeficiency. J Allergy Clin Im-munol 2004;114(2):415–21.

103. Lee AH, Levinson AI, Schumacher HR Jr. Hypogammaglobulinemia and rheu-matic disease. Semin Arthritis Rheum 1993;22(4):252–64.

104. Swierkot J, Lewandowicz-Uszynska A, Chlebicki A, et al. Rheumatoid arthritis in a patient with common variable immunodeficiency: difficulty in diagnosis and therapy. Clin Rheumatol 2006;25(1):92–4.

105. Resnick ES, Cunningham-Rundles C. The many faces of the clinical picture of common variable immune deficiency. Curr Opin Allergy Clin Immunol 2012; 12(6):595–601.

106. Jin R, Kaneko H, Suzuki H, et al. Age-related changes in BAFF and APRIL pro-files and upregulation of BAFF and APRIL expression in patients with primary antibody deficiency. Int J Mol Med 2008;21(2):233–8.

107. Wehr C, Eibel H, Masilamani M, et al. A new CD21low B cell population in the peripheral blood of patients with SLE. Clin Immunol 2004;113(2):161–71.

108. Park J, Munagala I, Xu H, et al. Interferon signature in the blood in inflammatory common variable immune deficiency. PLoS One 2013;8(9):e74893.

109. Gathmann B, Mahlaoui N, CEREDIH, et al. Clinical picture and treatment of 2212 patients with common variable immunodeficiency. J Allergy Clin Immunol 2014; 134(1):116–26.

110. Luzi G, Zullo A, Iebba F, et al. Duodenal pathology and clinical-immunological implications in common variable immunodeficiency patients. Am J Gastroen-terol 2003;98(1):118–21.

111. Malamut G, Verkarre V, Suarez F, et al. The enteropathy associated with common variable immunodeficiency: the delineated frontiers with celiac disease. Am J Gastroenterol 2010;105(10):2262–75.

112. Teahon K, Webster AD, Price AB, et al. Studies on the enteropathy associated with primary hypogammaglobulinaemia. Gut 1994;35(9):1244–9.

113. Biagi F, Bianchi PI, Zilli A, et al. The significance of duodenal mucosal atrophy in patients with common variable immunodeficiency: a clinical and histopathologic study. Am J Clin Pathol 2012;138(2):185–9.

114. Venhoff N, Emmerich F, Neagu M, et al. The role of HLA DQ2 and DQ8 in dis-secting celiac-like disease in common variable immunodeficiency. J Clin Immu-nol 2013;33(5):909–16.

115. Shulzhenko N, Morgun A, Hsiao W, et al. Crosstalk between B lymphocytes, microbiota and the intestinal epithelium governs immunity versus metabolism in the gut. Nat Med 2011;17(12):1585–93.

116. Mannon PJ, Fuss IJ, Dill S, et al. Excess IL-12 but not IL-23 accompanies the inflammatory bowel disease associated with common variable immunodeficiency. Gastroenterology 2006;131(3):748–56.

117. Lo B, Zhang K, Lu W, et al. Patients with LRBA deficiency show CTLA4 loss and immune dysregulation responsive to abatacept therapy. Science 2015; 359(6246):436–40.

118. Orange JS, Glessner JT, Resnick E, et al. Genome-wide association identifies diverse causes of common variable immunodeficiency. J Allergy Clin Immunol 2011;127(6):1360–7.e6.

119. Shi XZ, Sarna SK. Gene therapy of Cav1.2 channel with VIP and VIP receptor agonists and antagonists: a novel approach to designing promotility and anti-motility agents. Am J Physiol Gastrointest Liver Physiol 2008;295(1):G187–96.

120. Maglione PJ, Ko HM, Beasley MB, et al. Tertiary lymphoid neogenesis is a component of pulmonary lymphoid hyperplasia in patients with common variable immunodeficiency. J Allergy Clin Immunol 2014;133(2):535–42.

121. Randall TD. Bronchus-associated lymphoid tissue (BALT) structure and function. Adv Immunol 2010;107:187–241.

122. Baris S, Schulze I, Ozen A, et al. Clinical heterogeneity of immunodysregulation, polyendocrinopathy, enteropathy, X-linked: pulmonary involvement as a nonclassical disease manifestation. J Clin Immunol 2014;34(6):601–6.

123. Saunders BM, Britton WJ. Life and death in the granuloma: immunopathology of tuberculosis. Immunol Cell Biol 2007;85(2):103–11.

124. Mullighan CG, Fanning GC, Chapel HM, et al. TNF and lymphotoxin-alpha polymorphisms associated with common variable immunodeficiency: role in the pathogenesis of granulomatous disease. J Immunol 1997;159(12): 6236–41.

125. Wheat WH, Cool CD, Morimoto Y, et al. Possible role of human herpesvirus 8 in the lymphoproliferative disorders in common variable immunodeficiency. J Exp Med 2005;202(4):479–84.

126. Prasse A, Kayser G, Warnatz K. Common variable immunodeficiency-associated granulomatous and interstitial lung disease. Curr Opin Pulm Med 2013;19(5):503–9.

127. Fuss IJ, Friend J, Yang Z, et al. Nodular regenerative hyperplasia in common variable immunodeficiency. J Clin Immunol 2013;33(4):748–58.

128. Ward C, Lucas M, Piris J, et al. Abnormal liver function in common variable immunodeficiency disorders due to nodular regenerative hyperplasia. Clin Exp Immunol 2008;153(3):331–7.

129. Hartleb M, Gutkowski K, Milkiewicz P. Nodular regenerative hyperplasia: evolving concepts on underdiagnosed cause of portal hypertension. World J Gastroenterol 2011;17(11):1400–9.

130. Malamut G, Ziol M, Suarez F, et al. Nodular regenerative hyperplasia: the main liver disease in patients with primary hypogammaglobulinemia and hepatic abnormalities. J Hepatol 2008;48(1):74–82.

131. Wanless IR. Micronodular transformation (nodular regenerative hyperplasia) of the liver: a report of 64 cases among 2,500 autopsies and a new classification of benign hepatocellular nodules. Hepatology 1990;11(5):787–97.

132. Nakanuma Y. Nodular regenerative hyperplasia of the liver: retrospective survey in autopsy series. J Clin Gastroenterol 1990;12(4):460–5.

133. Reshamwala PA, Kleiner DE, Heller T. Nodular regenerative hyperplasia: not all nodules are created equal. Hepatology 2006;44(1):7–14.
134. Ziol M, Poirel H, Kountchou GN, et al. Intrasinusoidal cytotoxic CD8+ T cells in nodular regenerative hyperplasia of the liver. Hum Pathol 2004;35(10):1241–51.
135. Kiyuna A, Sunagawa T, Hokama A, et al. Nodular regenerative hyperplasia of the liver and Castleman's disease: potential role of interleukin-6. Dig Dis Sci 2005; 50(2):314–6.
136. Klein R, Goller S, Bianchi L. Nodular regenerative hyperplasia (NRH) of the liver–a manifestation of 'organ-specific antiphospholipid syndrome'? Immunobiology 2003;207(1):51–7.
137. Barzaghi F, Passerini L, Bacchetta R. Immune dysregulation, polyendocrinopathy, enteropathy, x-linked syndrome: a paradigm of immunodeficiency with autoimmunity. Front Immunol 2012;3:211.
138. Kluger N, Ranki A, Krohn K. APECED: is this a model for failure of T cell and B cell tolerance? Front Immunol 2012;3:232.
139. Tison BE, Nicholas SK, Abramson SL, et al. Autoimmunity in a cohort of 130 pediatric patients with partial DiGeorge syndrome. J Allergy Clin Immunol 2011; 128(5):1115–7.e1–3.
140. McLean-Tooke A, Barge D, Spickett GP, et al. Immunologic defects in 22q11.2 deletion syndrome. J Allergy Clin Immunol 2008;122(2):362–7, 367.e1–4.
141. Diehl L, Den Boer AT, van der Voort EI, et al. The role of CD40 in peripheral T cell tolerance and immunity. J Mol Med (Berlin, Germany) 2000;78(7):363–71.
142. Imai K, Slupphaug G, Lee WI, et al. Human uracil-DNA glycosylase deficiency associated with profoundly impaired immunoglobulin class-switch recombination. Nat Immunol 2003;4(10):1023–8.
143. Hanson EP, Monaco-Shawver L, Solt LA, et al. Hypomorphic nuclear factor-kappaB essential modulator mutation database and reconstitution system identifies phenotypic and immunologic diversity. J Allergy Clin Immunol 2008;122(6): 1169–77.e16.
144. Yoshioka T, Nishikomori R, Hara J, et al. Autosomal dominant anhidrotic ectodermal dysplasia with immunodeficiency caused by a novel NFKBIA mutation, p.Ser36Tyr, presents with mild ectodermal dysplasia and non-infectious systemic inflammation. J Clin Immunol 2013;33(7):1165–74.
145. Hernandez-Trujillo VP, Scalchunes C, Cunningham-Rundles C, et al. Autoimmunity and inflammation in X-linked agammaglobulinemia. J Clin Immunol 2014; 34(6):627–32.
146. Cleland SY, Siegel RM. Wiskott-Aldrich syndrome at the nexus of autoimmune and primary immunodeficiency diseases. FEBS Lett 2011;585(23):3710–4.
147. Abbott JK, Gelfand EW. Common Variable Immunodeficiency: Diagnosis, Management, and Treatment. Immunol Allergy Clin North Am 2015, in press.

Pulmonary Manifestations of Primary Immunodeficiency Disorders

Stephanie Nonas, MD

KEYWORDS

- Bronchiectasis • Interstitial lung disease • Primary immunodeficiency disease
- Common variable immune deficiency • Pulmonary complication

KEY POINTS

- Pulmonary complications of primary immunodeficiency disorders (PIDDs) are common and often unsuspected but significantly contribute to increased morbidity and mortality.
- In addition to lung infections, patients with PIDDs are at increased risk for other pulmonary complications, including asthma, bronchiectasis, interstitial lung disease, malignancy (lymphoma in particular), and autoimmune disease.
- A low threshold of suspicion is needed to ensure that pulmonary complications are caught early.
- Early diagnosis and treatment may affect the course of disease and improve patient outcomes.

INTRODUCTION

There are currently more than 200 recognized primary immunodeficiency disorders (PIDDs) ranging from deficiencies of humoral immunity with altered B-cell and antibody production to T-cell defects, phagocyte defects, and complement deficiencies, often with a degree of overlap. Pulmonary complications of PIDD are common and contribute significantly to morbidity and mortality in these patients. Recurrent pulmonary infections are often the first warning sign of PIDD and remain a leading cause of death from infectious causes in adults with PIDD. In addition, as survival from infectious disease improves, noninfectious pulmonary complications of PIDD, ranging from bronchiectasis and interstitial lung disease (ILD) to pulmonary malignancy and autoimmunity, are increasingly responsible for poor outcomes in PIDD. Early recognition and treatment of pulmonary complications may significantly alter disease

Division of Pulmonary and Critical Care Medicine, Oregon Health and Science University, 3181 Southwest Sam Jackson Park Road, UHN-67, Portland, OR 97239, USA
E-mail address: nonas@ohsu.edu

Immunol Allergy Clin N Am 35 (2015) 753–766
http://dx.doi.org/10.1016/j.iac.2015.07.004
0889-8561/15/$ – see front matter © 2015 Elsevier Inc. All rights reserved.
immunology.theclinics.com

progression and improve patient outcomes. This article reviews the primary patients with dysfunctional pulmonary complications of PIDD, with particular focus on early diagnosis and treatment.

PULMONARY INFECTIOUS COMPLICATIONS OF PRIMARY IMMUNODEFICIENCY DISORDER

Pulmonary infections are a major manifestation of primary immune deficiency. The presence of 2 or more pneumonias in a year is one of the 10 general warning signs of PIDD (Modell Foundation)[1] and retrospective studies have identified pneumonia as the top presenting feature of PIDD.[2,3] Despite variable clinical presentation in PIDDs, an increased susceptibility to infections is a hallmark feature that unites them. Recurrent pulmonary infections, including pneumonia, lung abscess, and/or empyema formation, account for significant morbidity and mortality in PIDD, accounting for 29% to 44% of deaths. The specific organisms involved in pulmonary infection vary by defect in immunity, with encapsulated organisms being typical pathogens in patients with deficient humoral immunity, and infections with fungal organisms being more typical of cellular deficiencies. Patients with dysfunctional phagocytes are particularly at risk for necrotizing pneumonias and lung abscesses, because of failure to effectively kill organisms such as *Staphylococcus aureus* and *Klebsiella pneumoniae*. A brief summary of the primary pulmonary infections in PIDD is provided in **Table 1**.

Infections in PIDD may sometimes be masked by other chronic symptoms, such as fever and adenopathy in patients with common variable immune deficiency (CVID) with lymphoproliferative disorder, thus symptoms such as new productive cough, change in sputum, and increased dyspnea should prompt an infectious evaluation with chest radiograph (CXR), sputum culture, and basic blood work as first-pass testing. Early recognition and treatment of acute infections is key to preventing severe infections and sepsis, which remain significant causes of mortality in these patients. However, the advent of widespread immunoglobulin replacement therapy has significantly decreased the prevalence of severe infections and death from infection causes in patients with CVID, X-linked agammaglobulinemia (XLA), and other disorders of humoral immunity.

NONINFECTIOUS COMPLICATIONS OF PRIMARY IMMUNODEFICIENCY DISORDER

The mortality from infectious complications of PIDD has significantly decreased in the past several decades, following the widespread standard use of immunoglobulin replacement therapy starting in the 1980s.[4,5] With this increased longevity came an increasing prevalence in, and mortality from, noninfectious complications in PIDD. In short, patients now live long enough to develop chronic noninfectious complications, particularly in the lungs. Noninfectious complications of PIDD, including bronchiectasis, ILD, pulmonary malignancy, and autoimmunity, have become the major cause of mortality in these patients and are responsible for the 11-fold increased risk of death in patients with noninfectious complications versus infectious complications of PIDD, an effect that is largely attributed to lymphoma, chronic lung disease, and hepatitis.[4] Although mortality from lower respiratory tract infections remains significant at 29% to 44%,[6,7] death caused by respiratory failure from chronic lung disease accounts for 30% to 36%[4,5] of the mortality in PIDD, whereas the prevalence of malignancies is 10% to 20% and accounts for 6% to 10% of mortality.[5,8] **Table 1** provides an overview of the common infectious and noninfectious complications of PIDDS. A brief summary of the typical clinical presentation as well as

Table 1
Infectious and Noninfectious Pulmonary Complications of PIDD

Primary Immunodeficiency	Pulmonary Infection	Noninfectious Pulmonary Complication

Deficiencies of humoral immunity [B-cell/antibody disorders] 50%–60% of primary immunodeficiencies Examples:
• Selective IgA deficiency
• CVID
• XLA
	Recurrent pneumonia with encapsulated and atypical organisms
	• *Streptococcus pneumoniae*
	• *Haemophilus influenzae*
	• *Neisseria*
	• *Mycoplasma* sp
	• Enteroviruses
		• Airway disease
		  ○ Asthma (in IgA deficiency)
		  ○ Bronchiectasis
		• ILD
		  ○ Lymphocytic interstitial pneumonitis
		  ○ OP
		  ○ GLILD (in CVID)
		• Lymphoma
		  ○ Non-Hodgkin lymphoma
		  ○ Hodgkin disease
		• Autoimmunity
		  ○ Immune thrombocytopenic purpura
		  ○ Autoimmune hemolytic anemia
		  ○ Rheumatoid arthritis
		  ○ Sjögren
		  ○ SLE
		  ○ Vasculitis

Phagocyte disorders 10%–15% of primary immunodeficiencies Examples:
• Chronic granulomatous disease
• Lymphocyte adhesion defect
• Chédiak-Higashi syndrome
	• Recurrent pulmonary infections, especially necrotizing pneumonia, lung abscess, and empyema, with bacterial and fungal organisms.
	  ○ *S aureus*
	  ○ *Klebsiella*
	  ○ *Burkholderia cepacia*
	  ○ *Serratia marcescens*
	  ○ *Aspergillus* sp
	  ○ *Nocardia*
		• Autoimmunity
		  ○ Antiphospholipid syndrome
		• ILD (CGD)

Deficiencies of cellular immunity 5%–10% of primary immunodeficiencies Examples:
• Wiskott-Aldrich syndrome,
• Di George syndrome
• X-linked lymphoproliferative syndrome
	• Recurrent pulmonary infections with:
	  ○ *Pseudomonas*
	  ○ Haemophilus
	  ○ Pneumococcus
	  ○ *Pneumocystis jiroveci*
	  ○ *Aspergillus* sp
	  ○ *Candida* sp
	  ○ CMV
	  ○ EBV
	  ○ Herpes virus
	  ○ Varicella
	  ○ Mycobacteria
		• Airway disease
		  ○ Bronchiectasis
		  ○ Bronchiolitis obliterans
		• Lymphoma

(continued on next page)

Table 1		
(continued)		
Primary Immunodeficiency	**Pulmonary Infection**	**Noninfectious Pulmonary Complication**
Combined humoral + cellular deficiency ~20% of primary immunodeficiencies Examples: • SCID • AT	Opportunistic infections, early in life. • CMV • Mucocutaneous candidiasis • P jiroveci • Mycobacteria • Invasive fungal (eg, aspergillus)	• ILD (in AT) • Lymphoma, leukemia (in AT)
Complement deficiencies ~2% of primary immunodeficiencies	Increased risk of respiratory tract infection, particularly from encapsulated organisms • S pneumoniae • H influenzae • Neisseria meningitidis	• Autoimmunity ○ SLE ○ Vasculitis

Abbreviations: AT, ataxia-telangiectasia; CGD, chronic granulomatous disease; CMV, cytomegalovirus; CVID, common variable immune deficiency; EBV, Epstein-Barr virus; GLILD, granulomatous-lymphocytic ILD; Ig, immunoglobulin; OP, organizing pneumonia; SCID, severe combined immunodeficiency; SLE, systemic lupus erythematosus; XLA, X-linked agammaglobulinemia.

pulmonary function test (PFT) and imaging findings for the common pulmonary complications of PIDD are presented in **Table 2**.

OBSTRUCTIVE AIRWAY DISEASE AND BRONCHIECTASIS

Obstructive airway disease, including asthma, bronchiolitis, and bronchiectasis, is extremely common in primary immunodeficiency. Obstructive spirometry is noted in 50% to 94% of patients.[9] Asthma is particularly common in patients with antibody deficiency, with rates between 15% and 42% of patients with CVID, selective immunoglobulin (Ig) A deficiency, and XLA.[10,11] Patients may present with typical symptoms of cough, wheezing, dyspnea, or chest tightness, but the diagnosis of asthma is confirmed by the presence of reversible airflow obstruction on prebronchodilator/postbronchodilator spirometry or the presence of airway hyperreactivity, as measured by a methacholine provocation test or similar. Note that normal spirometry does not rule out asthma. Because patients with PIDD have a high risk for multiple pulmonary complications that may present with similar symptoms (cough, dyspnea), spirometry is essential in the diagnosis of airway disease.

Bronchiectasis

Bronchiectasis is the permanent dilatation of bronchi, and bronchiolectasis is the permanent dilatation of bronchioli, although the distinction is often not made between dilatation of the large and small airways.[12] These abnormal, dilated airways are characterized by mucus hypersecretion and impaired mucociliary clearance, which impede the normal mechanisms by which the lungs clear pathogens. Patients with PIDD, particularly those with antibody deficiencies, are at markedly increased risk for developing bronchiectasis, particularly in CVID, in which the prevalence of bronchiectasis is greater than 70%.[13]

Bronchiectasis develops in PIDD because of the recurrent cycle of pulmonary infection, airway inflammation with consequent scarring and dilatation, and impaired bacterial clearance, which in turn leads to recurrent infection. In PIDD, increased susceptibility to pulmonary infection triggers and perpetuates this cycle. Thus the goals of therapy for bronchiectasis in PIDD include the early use of immunoglobulin replacement as well as traditional treatments for bronchiectasis designed to decrease infection and improve airway clearance.

Diagnosis

PFTs in bronchiectasis typically demonstrate obstruction, with a reduced forced expiratory volume in 1 second (FEV_1)/forced vital capacity (FVC) ratio and a reduced FEV_1. The obstruction may be reversible, in the presence of concomitant asthma, or irreversible. Imaging is the gold standard in diagnosing bronchiectasis. Findings of airway thickening and dilated bronchi may be seen on CXR with classic tram-track appearance (**Fig. 1**), but may be subtle and missed on CXR until significant dilatation has occurred. High-resolution computed tomography (HRCT) is far superior to CXR in detecting bronchial abnormalities, particularly before irreversible damage has been done. HRCT shows bronchiectasis and bronchiolectasis more clearly than plain CXR, with dilated airways seen in the lung periphery (**Fig. 2**, left) or the classic solitaire-ring sign, in which the cross-sectional diameter of the bronchiectatic airway is greater than 1.5 times that of the accompanying blood vessel (**Fig. 2**, right). Other common radiographic and computed tomography (CT) findings in bronchiectasis include airway thickening, mucus plugging, and tree-in-bud nodular opacities, reflecting chronic infection and poor clearance of secretions that are its hallmark features.

Unfortunately bronchiectasis often goes undiagnosed until permanent lung damage has occurred. Symptoms of dyspnea and daily productive cough are often attributed to chronic bronchitis/chronic obstructive pulmonary disease (COPD) or asthma and a CXR may not be obtained. Because of the significant delay in diagnosis of PIDD in many adults, which may be up to 4 to 5 years for CVID,[3] undiagnosed patients may develop bronchiectasis and permanent structural lung damage caused by years of recurrent respiratory infections long before their PIDD comes to light.

Treatment

Treatment of bronchiectasis focuses on (1) improving mucus clearance, (2) decreasing infection, and (3) decreasing inflammation.[14] Although mucus clearance has not been shown to affect mortality in clinical studies, regular airway clearance therapy is safe and does improve respiratory quality of life, exercise tolerance, sputum production, and hyperinflation. The addition of inhaled hypertonic saline to chest physiotherapy, meant to increase mucus water and decrease sputum viscosity, improves obstruction and increases FEV_1; however, other inhaled agents, such as mannitol and N-acetyl-cysteine, have not yet been shown to be helpful in controlled clinical trials. Note that recombinant DNase, which is an effective mainstay of therapy for bronchiectasis in cystic fibrosis, is potentially harmful in non–cystic fibrosis bronchiectasis, worsening FEV_1, and should not be used in patients with PIDD with bronchiectasis.

Antibiotics are a mainstay of treatment of many patients with PIDD, and several recent studies have shown significantly decreased rates of exacerbation of bronchiectasis and improved respiratory quality of life with chronic macrolide antibiotics (azithromycin, erythromycin). It remains unclear how much of this protective effect of macrolides is caused by immunomodulatory rather than antimicrobial properties of macrolides and there remain concerns for their long-term use, including the development of macrolide-resistant bacteria, particularly macrolide-resistant mycobacteria.

Table 2
Noninfectious Pulmonary Disease in PIDD: Clinical Presentation, PFT, and Imaging Findings

Pulmonary Complication	Symptoms	PFTs	Imaging

Bronchiectasis	• Chronic cough
	  ○ Copious mucopurulent sputum
	  ○ Hemoptysis
	• Dyspnea
	• Wheeze
	• Chest pain/tightness
		• Spirometry often shows obstruction, with decreased FEV_1/FVC ratio
		• Reversible obstruction after bronchodilator may be seen in 40% of patients
		• Airway hyperreactivity on methacholine challenge
			Typical features of CXR or CT chest:
			• Dilatation of bronchi and bronchioli (tram-track signs on CXR)
			  ○ Airway lumen >1.5× larger than adjacent blood vessel
			  ○ Lack of tapering of airways in the periphery
			  ○ Cystic spaces near the end of bronchi
			• Airway thickening
			• Mucus plugging of airways

ILD	• Progressive exertional dyspnea • Cough ○ Typically dry/nonproductive • Chest tightness	• PFTs are frequently abnormal • Spirometry is the least sensitive, but often suggests restrictive physiology • Lung volume testing may be normal but often shows restriction • DLCO testing is the most sensitive (although not specific) test. DLCO testing often shows impaired gas exchange, often the first PFT abnormality seen • 6-min walk test may show exertional desaturation	Typical features of ILD include the presence of diffuse ground-glass opacities with or without reticulation (indicates fibrosis) on chest radiograph and chest CT Findings suggestive of specific ILDs include: LIP • Bilateral ground-glass opacities with a diffuse or lower lung predominance • Septal thickening • Thin-walled cysts OP • Patchy consolidation or nodules in a bilateral peripheral and peribronchovascular distribution GLILD: combines features of granulomatous disease, LIP, and follicular bronchiolitis, which may include: • Hilar/mediastinal adenopathy • Lower lobe predominant reticulation • Diffuse ground glass (±cysts) • Bilateral centrilobular nodules • Bronchovascular and interlobular septal thickening • Fibrosis (in severe cases)
Asthma	Intermittent symptoms of: • Dyspnea • Dry cough • Wheezing, or • Chest tightness	• Abnormal spirometry showing reversible airflow obstruction, or • Normal spirometry[a] with airways hyperreactivity shown on methacholine challenge testing	CXR and CT chest are often normal, but may show airway thickening or hyperinflation

Bronchiolitis obliterans	• Exertional dyspnea • Cough • Chest tightness	Spirometry usually shows obstruction Lung volume testing: • Air trapping, with or without hyperinflation DLCO may be decreased, indicating a gas transfer abnormality	CXR is usually normal. In advanced bronchiolitis obliterans, there may be air trapping with hyperinflation or increase reticular markings seen on radiograph CT chest: • Mosaic attenuation indicates air trapping on expiratory-phase CT chest • Bronchial thickening

Pulmonary lymphoma	Patients may present with nonspecific pulmonary symptoms such as mild dyspnea, wheeze, cough, chest tightness, or systemic symptoms of fevers, weight loss, and night sweats
	~50% of patients are asymptomatic at the time of diagnosis
		PFTs are often normal at the time of diagnosis[b]
		A minority of patients with diffuse bilateral disease on presentation may have evidence of restriction and gas transfer abnormalities on PFT
			CXR
			• Paratracheal, hilar, and mediastinal lymphadenopathy, often presenting as a widened mediastinum
			• Parenchymal mass
			  ○ Often peripheral/pleural based
			  ○ With or without cavitation
			• Pleural effusion
			• Anterior mediastinal mass (seen on lateral CXR)
			CT chest (more sensitive than CXR)
			• Intraparenchymal pulmonary nodules, masses, or masslike consolidation
			  ○ Often peripheral/pleural based
			  ○ Often with air bronchogram or frank cavitation
			• Anterior mediastinal mass
			• Peribronchovascular thickening
			• Paratracheal, hilar, and/or mediastinal adenopathy
			• Pleural effusions
			• <10% with diffuse reticulonodular opacities

Abbreviations: CT, computed tomography; CXR, chest radiograph; DLCO, diffusion capacity for carbon monoxide; FEV$_1$, forced expiratory volume in 1 second; FVC, force vital capacity; LIP, lymphocytic interstitial pneumonia; OP, organizing pneumonia.

[a] Normal spirometry does not rule out asthma.
[b] Treatment of lymphoma with radiation or chemotherapy may result in diminished lung function with restriction and reduced gas transfer.

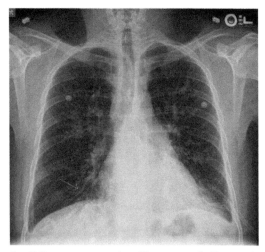

Fig. 1. Bronchiectasis: CXR, posteroanterior. The arrow indicates the classic tram-track appearance.

New studies are underway evaluating the efficacy of inhalational antibiotics, including colistin and aztreonam, to reduce airway bacterial load, inflammation, and exacerbations, while minimizing systemic absorption and toxicity.

Ultimately, some patients with bronchiectasis may benefit from inhaled corticosteroids, particularly those with concomitant asthma or COPD. However, given the increased risk of pneumonia reported in patients with non-PIDD COPD treated with daily inhaled corticosteroids, a risk/benefit discussion is recommended before initiating treatment and close follow-up is recommended while on treatment.

In addition, and specifically for patients with antibody deficiency, lifelong immunoglobulin therapy, using intravenous immunoglobulin (IVIG) or subcutaneous immunoglobulin (SCIG), prevents serious bacterial infections such as pneumonia and sepsis, and is one of the main reasons for the improved mortality in recent years. Newer studies suggest that the use of higher immunoglobulin trough targets (650–1000 mg/dL, which more accurately mimics normal physiologic levels, rather than

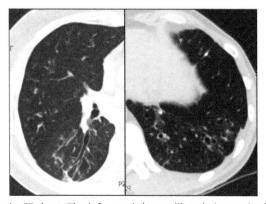

Fig. 2. Bronchiectasis: CT chest. The left panel shows dilated airways in the lung periphery, and the right panel shows the classic solitaire-ring sign.

the traditional 600 mL/dL) may slow or prevent the progression of chronic lung disease, including bronchiectasis.[15] Larger studies are underway, but perhaps the aggressive use of higher-dose immunoglobulin can effectively break the cycle of infection and chronic inflammation at the heart of bronchiectasis.

PARENCHYMAL/INTERSTITIAL LUNG DISEASE IN PRIMARY IMMUNODEFICIENCY DISORDER

Nearly 20% of patients with symptomatic antibody deficiency develop an ILD; a rate that is more than 200-fold higher than in the general population.[16,17] Patients with ILD are more likely to have CVID or other humoral deficiency, be older than 40 years, and to have a prior history of recurrent infections. The role of recurrent infections in causing ILD in this population is still being explored; however, one small study observed clinical and radiographic improvement in ILD in 28% of patients after IVIG therapy,[16] suggesting a possible contributing role for chronic infection.

The most common types of ILD in humoral deficiency are organizing pneumonia (OP; formerly called bronchiolitis obliterans organizing pneumonia or BOOP); lymphocytic interstitial pneumonia (LIP); and, in patients with CVID, granulomatous and lymphocytic ILD (GLILD). On HRCT of the chest, OP typically presents as persistent or migrating peribronchial or peripheral consolidation, whereas LIP is characterized by diffuse, bilateral ground-glass opacities, frequently with thin-walled cysts in a perivascular distribution. OP is unusual among ILDs because it typically responds well to treatment with high-dose corticosteroids followed by a slow taper. In contrast, there are few supportive data to show significant improvement in LIP with corticosteroids or other immune suppressants, although with worsening disease a trial of therapy is often initiated.

GLILD is a unique interstitial disease associated with CVID, with a prevalence of 10% to 15%. Characterized by granulomas as well as findings of follicular bronchiolitis, lymphoid hyperplasia, and LIP, GLILD is likely a pulmonary manifestation of systemic lymphoproliferative disorder. However, with granulomas and commonly a peribronchial pattern on imaging, GLILD is often misdiagnosed as sarcoidosis, despite being a distinct clinical entity with a significantly worse prognosis.[18] Randomized clinical trials of treatments in GLILD are lacking, and patients are often treated with high-dose corticosteroids or other immunosuppressives with mixed benefit and often harm. Recently, retrospective analyses have shown improvement in radiographic and PFT abnormalities in patients with CVID and GLILD treated with a combination of rituximab and azathioprine. In the absence of other effective therapy, and given the significant increase in mortality associated with GLILD, new prospective studies are urgently needed.

Other forms of ILD, including nonspecific pneumonitis (NSIP) and usual interstitial pneumonitis (UIP), have also been reported in patients with humoral deficiency, although they are less common than OP, LIP, or GLILD. NSIP and UIP share certain radiographic features: a subpleural reticulation, ground glass, and eventually traction bronchiectasis; however, NSIP shows more homogeneous involvement of the lungs and more extensive ground glass versus the heterogenous and lower lobe predominance of UIP. In addition, the presence of honeycombing on CT is nearly always diagnostic for UIP. As with many ILDs, treatment options for NSIP and UIP are limited. Trials of high-dose corticosteroids and steroid-sparing immunomodulatory drugs are typically used in NSIP with worsening lung function, but supporting data are limited. Conversely, in UIP multiple studies have now shown increased harm and no benefit with treatment with corticosteroids alone and in combination with immunosuppressive medications (such as azathioprine), and current recommendations are to avoid these therapies. Recently, 2 antifibrotic drugs (pirfenidone and nintedanib) have been approved in the United States specifically for the treatment of idiopathic pulmonary fibrosis; however, it remains unclear what role, if any, these drugs may have in the treatment of PIDD-related ILD.

Ataxia-telangiectasia (AT) is also associated with a high prevalence of ILD, with 25% of patients developing ILD.[19] Compared with patients with disorders of humoral immunity, patients with AT are younger and do not typically have evidence of preceding lung infection before the development of lung disease. Reported CT findings in AT did not meet diagnostic criteria for specific ILD, such as UIP or NSIP, but included bilateral septal thickening and interstitial and interlobar opacities. ILD in AT is associated with a significant increase in mortality, and 75% of patients died within 2 years of onset of lung disease. Notably, in this albeit small retrospective study, corticosteroids seemed to have a significant beneficial effect, with radiographic improvement and decreased mortality to 28% at 2 years.

The presence of ILD in PIDD increases mortality but early treatment may improve outcomes in certain diseases. With the high prevalence of ILD in AT, CVID, and other humoral deficiency states, clinicians must be vigilant in evaluating patients who present with typical symptoms of nonproductive cough, insidious onset of exertional dyspnea, hypoxemia, crackles, or clubbing on examination. PFTs can be useful in detecting restrictive pulmonary physiology, which is suggested by a decreased FVC with a high or normal FEV_1/FVC ratio on spirometry or more formally diagnosed using dedicated lung volume testing. Diffusion capacity for carbon monoxide (DLCO) testing can be helpful in diagnosing ILD, and typically is decreased, reflecting a loss in alveolar-capillary gas transfer surface. The greater the lung involvement with ILD, the greater the defect in gas transfer. Note that DLCO testing is very sensitive, but not specific, for ILD and may also be decreased in emphysema and pulmonary hypertension.

Although symptoms and PFTs can point to pulmonary parenchymal pathology HRCT is the main diagnostic tool for detecting ILD. Chest HRCT plays a crucial role in the diagnosis and management of ILD in PIDD, allowing the detection of findings too subtle to be seen on plain CXR and improved three-dimensional imaging of findings that help differentiate the different ILDs. Many patients with a classic radiographic presentation for a specific ILD (honeycombing in UIP, the presence of ground glass and cysts in LIP) do not get a lung biopsy because it would not change management. However, a diagnostic lung biopsy may be performed when the diagnosis is in question or when malignancy is on the differential.

Bronchoscopic biopsies are generally inadequate for the diagnosis of parenchymal lung disease. The main utility of bronchoscopy in these patients is in ruling out infectious and other causes of abnormal lung findings, such as Pneumocystis jiroveci or pulmonary lymphoma. A surgical lung biopsy, either an open lung biopsy or the minimally invasive video-assisted thoracoscopic technique, may be needed to obtain a large enough tissue sample for accurate diagnosis. Compared with bronchoscopic biopsies, surgical lung biopsies can give much larger tissue samples, which is useful because there may often be different histologic patterns in the same biopsy. As always, the risks and benefits of lung biopsy must be weighed and the question asked: will this result change the plan of therapy? Because many ILDs have no specific targeted therapy, if lung biopsy results will not change the plan for an empiric trial of high-dose corticosteroid treatment, it may be better to spare the patient an invasive and painful procedure.

A diagnosis of ILD often requires referral to a pulmonary specialist and is often made in conjunction with clinicians, radiologists, and pathologists. Treatment, even empiric, should be discussed with the patient's primary clinician as well as pulmonary and immunology specialists. In addition to targeted therapies for ILD, all patients with more than mild pulmonary involvement on PFT or CT should be screened for oxygen therapy with desaturation testing at rest, with exercise, and with sleep. Supplemental oxygen should be used to maintain oxygen saturation in the 88% to 95% range to avoid hypoxemia and hyperoxia. Referral to pulmonary rehabilitation can significantly improve functional status, exercise capacity, and quality of life.

MALIGNANCY

Malignancy is now one of the leading causes of death in patients with PIDD.[5,8,20] As clinicians do a better job preventing and treating infectious complications of primary immune deficiency, with immunoglobulin replacement and judicious use of antimicrobials, patients live long enough to develop, and die from, malignancy. Overall, patients with PIDD have a 5-fold greater risk of malignancy, largely caused by defective immune surveillance. However, this excess risk is almost entirely caused by 5 specific subgroups of PIDD: CVID, AT, Wiskott-Aldrich syndrome, severe combined immunodeficiency, and IgA deficiency. CVID alone carries a 30-fold to 400-fold increased risk for non-Hodgkin lymphoma compared with the general population. Lymphomas, both Hodgkin and non-Hodgkin lymphoma, are by far the most common malignancies in PIDD, accounting for 10% and 48.6% of cancers in patients with primary immunodeficiency, respectively. Although not always a specific pulmonary complication, lymphomas in PIDD are more likely to present in extranodal sites, including the lungs and gastrointestinal tract, and thus may present with respiratory complaints.

Perhaps the most difficult part of diagnosing lymphoma in patients with primary immune deficiency is the frequent overlap in symptoms between lymphoma and the underlying PIDD. Fevers, fatigue, weight loss, and adenopathy are common in PIDDs, especially CVID, because of infectious and noninfectious causes. Thus a lowered threshold of suspicion is required to suspect underlying malignancy, particularly in the presence of new findings on chest imaging. HRCT features for pulmonary lymphoma include peribronchovascular thickening or nodules, pleural effusion, patchy ground-glass airspace opacities, masslike consolidation (often pleural based), and hilar/mediastinal adenopathy. However, many of these features are nonspecific for lymphoma and patients with adenopathy and peribronchovascular nodules may be mistakenly given a clinical diagnosis of sarcoidosis, delaying diagnosis of their lymphomas. Thus, if there are radiographic findings and clinical suspicion for lymphoma, referral for bronchoscopy with transbronchial biopsy and/or needle aspirate can confirm the diagnosis using cytopathologic staining and flow cytometry for lymphoma markers.

Treatment of malignancy in PIDD is no different than in immunocompetent patients. Ongoing supportive immunoglobulin should be continued if indicated at baseline. However, the prognosis for malignancy in primary immunodeficiency is typically worse than for other patients, because of increased risk of infectious complications and further organ damage from chemotherapy.[5] Likewise, radiation therapy, a common adjunctive therapy for Hodgkin disease, is associated with acute radiation pneumonitis and chronic lung fibrosis, further contributing to pulmonary morbidity and mortality.

AUTOIMMUNITY IN PRIMARY IMMUNODEFICIENCY DISORDER

Autoimmunity is another, often undersuspected, complication of primary immunodeficiency, particularly in patients with humoral/antibody deficiencies. Approximate 25% of patients with CVID and IgA deficiency develop some form of autoimmunity.[21,22] In

CVID, the most common manifestations of autoimmune disease are autoimmune hemolytic anemia and immune thrombocytopenias; however, patients are also at higher risk for autoimmune connective tissue diseases such as rheumatoid arthritis (RA), Sjögren syndrome, systemic lupus erythematosus (SLE), and various types of vasculitis. Likewise, XLA is associated with juvenile RA and dermatomyositis, and IgA deficiency with RA, SLE, and immune thrombocytopenia. Complement deficiency is significantly associated with SLE, and chronic granulomatous disease, hyper-IgM syndrome, and Wiskott-Aldrich with inflammatory bowel disease (IBD).

The significance of autoimmune disease in a review of pulmonary complications of PIDDs is that autoimmune and connective tissue diseases are associated with increased rates of pulmonary complications themselves. For example, RA is significantly associated with airway diseases, including bronchiectasis and bronchiolitis, pleural disease, as well as ILDs (UIP>NSIP); Sjögren disease with ILD (NSIP>LIP); SLE with acute pneumonitis; and IBD with airway disease, ILD, and pulmonary vasculitis.

As discussed earlier, the presence of chronic lung disease, particularly ILD, significantly increases morbidity and mortality in PIDD. However, there is some evidence that autoimmune-associated ILDs may be more responsive to therapy than their idiopathic counterparts. In addition, therapies targeted at specific immune cell subsets, such as rituximab for B cell–mediated disease and anti–tumor necrosis factor therapies for IBD, may be better able to target the systemic and pulmonary complications of autoimmunity without the need for nonspecific immunosuppressive treatment with glucocorticoids.

SCREENING AND TESTING RECOMMENDATIONS

The clinician faced with a patient with known PIDD presenting with a new or worsening pulmonary complaint should have a low threshold for further evaluation, including CXR and sputum cultures for suspected acute pneumonia, spirometry if there is suspicion for asthma or bronchiectasis, and full PFTs (including spirometry, lung volume testing, and DLCO) if restrictive or infiltrative lung disease is suspected. Persistent symptoms of dyspnea, cough, wheezing, and hypoxemia should prompt more extensive testing, including full PFTs and HRCT if there is concern for ILD or malignancy.

Screening of asymptomatic patients is less straightforward. Of the common PIDDs, CVID has the most specific recommendations,[20] consisting of yearly screening with pulmonary function testing (including spirometry and DLCO) and chest CT initially and every 5 years. Other groups recommend PFTs and CXR only at the time of referral in patients without respiratory symptoms, but recommend screening with chest CT every 3 to 4 years or with any significant change in therapy.[21] The general recommendation is for the judicious use of chest CT, given the radiation dose in patients already at increased risk for malignancy. PFTs, particularly when lung volumes and DLCO are monitored, can noninvasively provide information about both obstructive and restrictive disease without radiation exposure.

OTHER POINTS
Smoking Cessation

In addition to the increase in risk for lung cancer and COPD/emphysema, tobacco use increases susceptibility to bacterial and mycobacterial lung infections. Tobacco smoke adversely affects ciliary function in the lower respiratory tract as well as antimicrobial function of leukocytes. In patients with existing lung disease, cigarette smoking may accelerate the development of obstruction and contribute to worsening symptoms. Early and aggressive counseling on the importance of avoiding tobacco is recommended in all patients with PIDD. Patients should be encouraged and supported aggressively in their efforts to quit.

Vaccine-Preventable Lung Disease

One final key issue in preventing pulmonary complications of PIDD is the use of vaccines. Yearly vaccination for influenza (with the inactivated killed vaccine) and age-appropriate pneumococcal pneumonia vaccination are generally recommended for patients with chronic lung disease, such as ILD or bronchiectasis. However, patients with defective humoral immunity may not be able to mount an adequate response to vaccination, rendering the vaccination useless. More importantly, the use of live vaccines (including the live-attenuate FluMist influenza vaccine) is contraindicated in most patients with primary immunodeficiency, as well as their household contacts. Formal guidelines for the vaccination of patients with primary immunodeficiency are available at the US Centers for Disease Control and Prevention (CDC) Web site (www.cdc.gov/vaccines). If in doubt, consulting the CDC guidelines or referral to immunologist is recommended. Patients treated with immunoglobulin replacement gain some immunity via passive antibodies from vaccinated donors.

SUMMARY

Pulmonary diseases ranging from infectious pneumonias, lung abscess, and empyema to structural lung diseases to malignancy significantly increase morbidity and mortality in primary immune deficiency. Treatment with supplemental immunoglobulin (IVIG or SCIG) and antimicrobials is beneficial in reducing infections but may be ineffective in preventing noninfectious complications, including ILD, malignancy, and autoimmune disease. A low threshold for suspecting pulmonary complications is necessary for the early diagnosis of pulmonary involvement in PIDD, before irreversible damage is done, to improve patient outcomes.

REFERENCES

1. Arkwright PD, Gennery AR. Ten warning signs of primary immunodeficiency: a new paradigm is needed for the 21st century. Ann N Y Acad Sci 2011;1238:7–14.
2. Rezaei N, Aghamohammadi A, Moin M, et al. Frequency and clinical manifestations of patients with primary immunodeficiency disorders in Iran: update from the Iranian Primary Immunodeficiency Registry. J Clin Immunol 2006;26:519–32.
3. Cunningham-Rundles C, Bodian C. Common variable immunodeficiency: clinical and immunological features of 248 patients. Clin Immunol 1999;92:34–48.
4. Resnick ES, Moshier EL, Godbold JH, et al. Morbidity and mortality in common variable immune deficiency over 4 decades. Blood 2012;119:1650–7.
5. Shapiro RS. Malignancies in the setting of primary immunodeficiency: implications for hematologists/oncologists. Am J Hematol 2011;86:48–55.
6. Al-Herz W, Moussa MAA. Survival and predictors of death among primary immunodeficient patients: a registry-based study. J Clin Immunol 2012;32:467–73.
7. Mir Saeid Ghazi B, Aghamohammadi A, Kouhi A, et al. Mortality in primary immunodeficient patients, registered in Iranian primary immunodeficiency registry. Iran J Allergy Asthma Immunol 2004;3:31–6.
8. Quinti I, Agostini C, Tabolli S, et al. Malignancies are the major cause of death in patients with adult onset common variable immunodeficiency. Blood 2012;120:1953–4.

9. Touw CM, van de Ven AA, de Jong PA, et al. Detection of pulmonary complications in common variable immunodeficiency. Pediatr Allergy Immunol 2009;21: 793–805.

10. Agondi RC, Barros MT, Rizzo LV, et al. Allergic asthma in patients with common variable immunodeficiency. Allergy 2010;65:510–5.

11. Özcan C, Metin A, Erkoçoğlu M, et al. Bronchial hyperreactivity in children with antibody deficiencies. Allergol Immunopathol (Madr) 2015;43:57–61.

12. Barker AF. Bronchiectasis. N Engl J Med 2002;346:1383–93.

13. Thickett KM, Kumararatne DS, Banerjee AK, et al. Common variable immune deficiency: respiratory manifestations, pulmonary function and high-resolution CT scan findings. QJM 2002;95:655–62.

14. Chalmers JD, Aliberti S, Blasi F. State of the art review: management of bronchiectasis in adults. Eur Respir J 2015. http://dx.doi.org/10.1183/09031936.00119114.

15. Kobrynski L. Subcutaneous immunoglobulin therapy: a new option for patients with primary immunodeficiency diseases. Biologics 2012;6:277–87.

16. Popa V, Colby TV, Reich SB. Pulmonary interstitial disease in Ig deficiency. Chest 2002;122:1594–603.

17. Bierry G, Boileau J, Barnig C, et al. Thoracic manifestations of primary humoral immunodeficiency: a comprehensive review. Radiographics 2009;29:1909–20.

18. Bates CA, Ellison MC, Lynch DA, et al. Granulomatous-lymphocytic lung disease shortens survival in common variable immunodeficiency. J Allergy Clin Immunol 2004;114:415–21.

19. Schroeder SA, Swift M, Sandoval C, et al. Interstitial lung disease in patients with ataxia-telangiectasia. Pediatr Pulmonol 2005;39:537–43.

20. Deane S, Selmi C, Naguwa SM, et al. Common variable immunodeficiency: etiological and treatment issues. Int Arch Allergy Immunol 2009;150:311–24.

21. Cunningham-Rundles C. How I treat common variable immune deficiency. Blood 2010;116:7–15.

22. Edwards E, Razvi S, Cunningham-Rundles C. IgA deficiency: clinical correlates and responses to pneumococcal vaccine. Clin Immunol 2004;111:93–7.

Primary Immunodeficiency Masquerading as Allergic Disease

Sanny K. Chan, MD, PhD*, Erwin W. Gelfand, MD

KEYWORDS

- Primary immune deficiency • Corticosteroids • Eczema • Elevated IgE
- Allergic disease

KEY POINTS

- Primary immune deficiencies (PIDs) are uncommon diseases, including several with overlapping clinical presentations to common allergic and autoimmune diseases.
- Early recognition and diagnosis of PIDs is critical.
- Immune suppression should be initiated judiciously because it can increase the susceptibility to life-threatening diseases in PID patients.

INTRODUCTION

Primary immune deficiencies (PIDs) are an uncommon heterogeneous group of diseases that result from fundamental defects in the proteins and cells that enable specific immune responses. Most are inherited and often appear in family members. Remarkably, many of these diseases do not demonstrate predictable clear-cut clinical patterns. For many, the hallmark is an increased susceptibility to infection; and different pathogens associate with different defects of the immune system. The true incidence and prevalence of these primary immunodeficiencies are unknown, but are estimated to be 1:10,000 to 1:2000 from registries in more than 40 countries.[1] This is likely an underestimation because many cases remain undiagnosed; a random telephone survey in the United States estimated the prevalence of all PIDs at 1:2000 to 1:800.[2] Early diagnosis of a PID has a significant bearing on outcome. For example, newborn screening for severe combined immune deficiency (SCID) has resulted in important early diagnoses and when treated with hematopoietic stem cell transplantation (HSCT) before 3.5 months of age, a 94% success rate can be achieved compared with older individuals with infections at the time of transplant (50%).[3]

Disclosures: Neither author has anything to disclose.
Division of Allergy and Immunology, Department of Pediatrics, National Jewish Health, 1400 Jackson Street, Denver, CO 80206, USA
* Corresponding author.
E-mail address: chans@njhealth.org

Immunol Allergy Clin N Am 35 (2015) 767–778
http://dx.doi.org/10.1016/j.iac.2015.07.008
0889-8561/15/$ – see front matter
immunology.theclinics.com

What is increasingly being recognized is that common allergic symptoms can also be manifestations of an underlying and severe immune deficiency (**Fig. 1**). The immune system relies on a complex balance of activation, to protect against invading pathogens, and control, to discriminate between self, nonself, and foreign matter. Hypersensitivity (allergic) reactions (eczema, allergic rhinitis, asthma, and food allergies) are exaggerated immune responses against specific allergens. Classic testing used to investigate allergic diseases often reveals increased immunoglobulin (Ig)E, peripheral blood eosinophilia, and immediate skin responses after percutaneous or intradermal injection. It is now clear that some of these PIDs do not manifest with a predominant susceptibility to infection, but rather present with what seems to be more common allergic symptoms or autoimmunity.[4] Recognition of these immunodeficiencies is important because their treatments are profoundly different than the treatments for an allergic condition, the latter often involving use of immunosuppressive therapies. In PID patients, further suppression of the immune system increases susceptibility to a life-threatening event, namely, infection. If the classic allergic triad includes increased IgE, eosinophilia, and eczema, then under this umbrella are a number of genetically defined PIDs that masquerade as allergy and warrant different therapeutic approaches (**Table 1**).

ALL THAT ITCHES IS NOT ALWAYS ECZEMA

Eczema is a complex, chronic, relapsing inflammatory skin disorder with a lifetime prevalence in the United States of 17%.[5] Interestingly, 80% have an elevated serum IgE.[6] It is the earliest part of the allergic march toward allergic rhinitis and asthma, with 66% of patients progressing to develop asthma plus at least 1 allergy by 3 years of age.[7]

Pathophysiology

Eczema and atopic dermatitis present early in infancy, usually between 1 and 6 months of age. Resolution occurs in 50% by adolescence, but factors that suggest a poorer prognosis include family medical history of eczema, early infantile disease, gender (female), coexistent allergic rhinitis, or asthma.[8] Although the exact mechanism remains unclear, breaks in the skin barrier lead to sensitization to allergens, increased IgE levels, and increased numbers of eosinophils.

PRIMARY IMMUNE DEFICIENCY PRESENTING WITH NEWBORN AND INFANT ECZEMA

Although a common condition, eczema in a newborn warrants a number of diagnostic considerations and concerns. Severe whole body dermatitis appearing as an

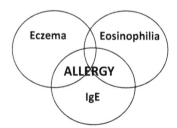

Fig. 1. The allergic triad. Allergic diseases share common factors with primary immunodeficiencies including skin rashes such as eczema, increased immunoglobulin (Ig)E, and eosinophilia.

Table 1 Phenotypic expression of eczema, eosinophilia, and increased IgE in primary immunodeficiency		
Eczema	**Eosinophilia**	**Increased IgE**
IPEX	IPEX	IPEX
Omenn	Omenn	Omenn
AD-HIES	AD-HIES	AD-HIES
AR-HIES	AR-HIES	AR-HIES
Wiskott-Adrich	—	—

Various primary immunodeficiencies have a predominance in manifestation of their disease.
  Abbreviations: AD-HIES, autosomal-dominant hyper-IgE syndrome; AR-HIES, autosomal recessive hyper-IgE syndrome; IG, immunoglobulin; IPEX, immune dysregulation, polyendocrinopathy, enteropathy, X-linked syndrome.

eczematous rash and loose stool/diarrhea may be mistaken as an atopic baby with food allergy. Clinicians should consider PIDs especially if standard interventions with topical steroids and changing formulas are helpful only transiently. PIDs may mimic allergic atopic patients.[4]

Human Immunodeficiency Virus

Infants with human immunodeficiency virus (HIV) infection (a secondary immunodeficiency) can present with eczematous rash, high IgE, and failure to thrive. It is one of the more common immunodeficiencies and should always be excluded when considering a PID. Virologic testing with HIV DNA polymerase or HIV RNA assays should be used.

Omenn Syndrome

Omenn syndrome is an inflammatory condition characterized by erythroderma, desquamatous alopecia, chronic diarrhea, failure to thrive, lymphedema, and hepatomegaly.[9] It was originally described in 1965 with reticuloendotheliosis and eosinophilia.[10] The prevalence is estimated at less than 1/1,000,000.[11] It is linked to SCID and presents in the first year of life, but the signs and symptoms evolve over time. These patients are highly susceptible to the infections that are typically seen in SCID patients.

Pathogenesis
There are no specific genetic defects for Omenn syndrome. It is an inflammatory phenotype of SCID that has been linked to mutations in the recombination-activating gene 1 (RAG1) or RAG2, RNA component of mitochondrial RNA processing endoribonuclease, adenosine deaminase, interleukin (IL)-2R, IL-7R, artemis-nuclease-DCLRE1C DNA ligase 4, and 22q11 microdeletion. It usually presents in an autosomal-recessive pattern. This is a "leaky" T/B-SCID phenotype where some T or B cells are present and suggestive of mutations that lead to impairment of the V(D)J DNA recombination involved in generating immunoglobulins as well as T-cell receptors.

Diagnosis
Omenn syndrome is characterized by clinical inflammation with abnormal T-cell populations. Lymphocyte phenotyping by flow cytometry show T-cell lymphopenia or oligoclonality that have impaired function. Typically, B cells are absent with loss of IgG, IgA, IgM, but increased serum IgE. Peripheral blood eosinophilia is also present. Skin biopsy of lesions show acanthosis and parakeratosis.

Differential diagnosis
In addition to Omenn syndrome, infants with severe eczematous dermatitis with diarrhea may not just be a severely atopic infant with food allergy, but consideration of other PIDs include an SCID patient with maternal T-cell engraftment syndrome causing graft versus host disease, infantile ichthyosis, histiocytosis, and hyper-IgE syndrome.

Management
Given the rarity of PIDs, unlike HIV, therapies have not been studied in large-scale clinical trials, but only in small series or case reports. Immunosuppressive treatment has been used in Omenn syndrome to control inflammation. Suppression can result in almost complete resolution of the dermatitis, alopecia, hepatosplenomegaly, and lymphadenopathy with significant weight gain.[12] Care should be taken to treat underlying infections and screening for opportunistic infections should be initiated before immune suppression, given the underlying SCID phenotype. To date, curative treatment and ultimate resolution requires HSCT.[13]

X-linked Immunodysregulation, Polyendocrinopathy, and Enteropathy

Infants with immune dysregulation, polyendocrinopathy, enteropathy, X-linked syndrome (IPEX) usually present with severe diarrhea owing to enteropathy, endocrinopathy usually manifesting as type 1 diabetes mellitus, and dermatitis (eczema, erythroderma). Other features may include hypothyroidism, autoimmune hemolytic anemia, thrombocytopenia, lymphadenopathy, hepatitis, and nephritis. IPEX was originally described in 1982[14] and the prevalence is estimated at less than 1 in 1,000,000[15] with only around 200 cases reported to date. Patients present in the first year of life and severity varies.

Pathogenesis
IPEX is an X-linked recessive disease caused by a mutation in the FoxP3 gene on chromosome Xp11. This transcription factor plays an important role in the development and function of T regulatory cells that are actively involved in suppressing the immune system and in self-tolerance.[16] These T regulatory cells (CD4$^+$25$^+$) control T- and B-cell inflammatory reactions. FoxP3 binds to the FOX-binding site within the IL-2 promoter and suppresses its activity.

Diagnosis
IPEX patients have elevated IgE, IgA, and peripheral blood eosinophilia. The diagnosis is often made after endoscopy. Enteric biopsy may reveal villous atrophy reminiscent of severe gastrointestinal graft versus host disease or autoimmune enteropathy (with the presence of antienterocyte, harmonin, and villin autoantibodies). Evaluation for IPEX should follow the diagnosis of infant-onset insulin-dependent diabetes mellitus. It is linked to type 1 diabetes mellitus (antibodies against insulin, pancreatic islet cells, or antiglutamate decarboxylase), thyroiditis (antithyroglobulin and antimicrosome peroxidase antibodies), and cytopenia (antiplatelet and antineutrophil antibodies, positive Coombs test). Lymphocyte subset phenotyping with flow cytometry shows loss of CD4$^+$25$^+$ T regulatory cells. Molecular diagnosis with identification of mutations in FoxP3 confirms IPEX and it can identify aberrant sequences that result in termination/frameshift/missense mutations. Location and identification of the mutation can help to stratify for progression and severity of disease.[17]

Differential diagnosis
The triad of endocrine dysfunction, enteropathy, and inflammatory eczema in infant males is suggestive of IPEX, although other diseases should be considered, including IPEX-like syndrome in CD25 mutations that affect both genders; STAT5b mutation;

ITCH syndrome, the Nedd4 family of HECT domain E3 ubiquitin ligase mutation; Schmidt syndrome/autoimmune polyendocrinopathy syndrome type 1; autoimmune polyendocrinopathy, candidiasis, ectodermal dystrophy; Wiskott–Aldrich; STAT1 (gain of function); X-linked autoimmune enteropathy; and X-linked thrombocytopenia.

Management

Supportive care (including parenteral nutrition, blood transfusions, and controlling diabetes) are the mainstays of treatment. High-dose corticosteroids, cyclosporine, tacrolimus, methotrexate, infliximab, and rituximab have been used. Sirolimus has been effective.[18] Allogeneic HSCT resulted in a rapid and sustained decrease in symptoms of enteropathy, eczema, and diabetes, which was accompanied by a decrease in the concentration of autoantibodies directed against pancreatic proteins.[19,20] HSCT for IPEX is still evolving and consultation with experts in bone marrow transplantation is important because reduced-intensity conditioning regimens using alemtuzumab, fludarabine, and melphalan may be beneficial.[21] Activation of the immune system makes symptoms, including blood glucose levels, more difficult to control. Extensive infectious and virology-based studies should be investigated and early treatment initiated.

Wiskott–Aldrich Syndrome

Infant males with severe diarrhea, eczema, and thrombocytopenia should be evaluated for Wiskott–Aldrich syndrome. Because of severe thrombocytopenia (which typically causes bloody diarrhea), most cases present with hemorrhagic manifestations of this syndrome yet eczematous skin lesions are readily visible. These males are prone to recurrent infections, with a component of autoimmunity in approximately 40% of cases. It was originally described in 1954,[22] and the prevalence is estimated at around 4 in 1,000,000.[23]

Pathogenesis

Wiskott–Aldrich syndrome is an X-linked recessive disease owing to hemizygous mutations in the Wiskott–Aldrich syndrome gene (Xp11.4-p11.21), coding for the Wiskott–Aldrich syndrome protein (WASp), which is exclusively expressed in hematopoietic cells and plays a critical role in the organization of the actin cytoskeleton. WASp is involved in T-cell actin reorganization,[24] coupling surface Ig and signal transduction for B-cell activation,[25] as well as natural killer (NK) cell cytotoxicity. All immune cells, B, NK, and T cells are affected, resulting in a combined phenotype.

Diagnosis

Wiskott–Aldrich syndrome has a typical triad of thrombocytopenia, eczema, and recurrent infections. These patients have elevated IgE, IgA, and eosinophilia. They have thrombocytopenia with reduced platelet size and a normal number of megakaryocytes, as well as impaired antibody production (mainly antipolysaccharide antibodies). The molecular diagnosis with loss of WASp confirms Wiskott–Aldrich syndrome. Genetic diagnosis to identify aberrant sequences that result in termination/frameshift/missense mutations may help to predict disease course and prenatal diagnosis should be considered in familial cases.

Differential diagnosis

Males with recurrent infections, eczema, and thrombocytopenia suggests Wiskott–Aldrich syndrome, but other syndromes to consider include Wiskott-Aldrich syndrome-2 (WAS2) caused by mutations in the WAS/WASL-interacting protein family member 1 (WIPF1) gene coding for a protein that stabilizes and prevents the degradation of WASp, acute or chronic idiopathic thrombocytopenia, and thrombocytopenia-absent radius syndrome.

Management

Patients with Wiskott–Aldrich syndrome may require intensive support with parenteral nutrition, blood transfusions, platelet transfusions, and intravenous immunoglobulin. Agonists of the thrombopoietin receptors (such as romiplostim and eltrombopag) have been used with some success. The only curative treatment to date is HSCT. The goal is to control the autoimmune manifestations and bleeding disorder, without further suppressing the immune system. Wiskott–Aldrich syndrome patients are prone to tumors (mainly B-cell lymphomas). Interesting in vivo reversions have been reported.[26,27] Gene therapy is being trialed in cases where there is no adequate HSCT match, but remains experimental.[28,29]

PIDS PRESENTING WITH EOSINOPHILIA, INCREASED IMMUNOGLOBULIN E, AND ECZEMA: IT MAY NOT JUST BE ATOPY

Autosomal-Dominant Hyper-immunoglobulin E Syndrome–Job Syndrome

Autosomal-dominant hyper-IgE syndrome (AD-HIES), also known as Job syndrome, characteristically features chronic eczema, recurrent staphylococcal skin infections, increased serum IgE, and eosinophilia. Patients usually have a distinctive coarse facial appearance, abnormal dentition with retained primary teeth, hyperextensibility of the joints, and bone fractures.[30] They are prone to infections: recurrent "cold" skin abscesses (lacking the classical feature of red, warm, tender abscesses filled with pus), pneumonia with pneumatocele formation, and mucocutaneous candidiasis (**Table 2**). Interestingly, many feel fine even during severe infections. HIES was

Table 2 AD-HIES and AR-HIES			
	AD-HIES	AR-HIES	
Gene Association	STAT3	DOCK8	TYK2
Mostly de novo mutations	X	—	—
Increased IgE	X	X	X
Eczema	X	X	X
Eosinophilia	X	X	X
Coarse facies	X	—	—
Skeletal abnormalities	X	—	—
Retained primary teeth	X	—	—
Hyperextensible joints	X	—	—
Pulmonary pneumatocele	X	—	—
Viral skin infections	—	X	X
Asthma	—	X	—
Food allergies	—	X	—
Decreased IgM	—	X	—
Mycobacterium susceptibility	—	—	X
Difficulty handling herpes simplex virus and Molluscum	—	X	X
CNS manifestations	—	X	X
Cerebral vascular malformations	—	X	X

The 2 predominant inherited forms of hyper-IgE syndrome have overlapping similarities, as well as distinct differences that can suggest the underlying genetic defect

Abbreviations: AD-HIES, autosomal-dominant hyper-IgE syndrome; AR-HIES, autosomal-recessive hyper-IgE syndrome; CNS, neurologic; IG, immunoglobulin.

originally described in 1966.[31] Serum IgE levels are often greater than 2000 IU/mL, eosinophilia often greater than 700 cells/mL, but patients usually lack any symptomatic allergic disease such as allergic rhinitis, food allergy, or anaphylaxis.

The overlapping clinical features with atopic patients led to clinical scoring criteria to assess the probability of AD-HIES. In 1999, the National Institutes of Health HIES scoring system was developed where a score of greater than 15 indicated that AD-HIES was likely owing to STAT3 deficiency.[32] This was further refined based on a total IgE concentration greater than 1000 IU/mL and a weighted score of clinical features so that a score greater than 30 predicts a STAT3 mutation.[33] Approximately 60% to 70% of cases are the result of a dominant-negative mutation in the signal transducer and activator of transcription 3 (STAT3) gene.[33] The etiology in the remaining 30% is unknown, and the prevalence is estimated between 1 and 9 in 100,000.[34]

Pathogenesis

A dominant-negative heterozygous mutation in STAT3 leads to AD-HIES. STAT3 is located at 17q21.31 and is critical in the signal transduction of a broad range of cytokines that act as transcription activators. Phosphorylation of tyrosine 705 leads to activation and the formation of homodimers or heterodimers, which then translocate to the cell nucleus. They respond to cytokines and growth factors including: interferons, epidermal growth factor, IL-5, IL-6, hepatocyte growth factor, leukemia inhibitory factor, bone morphogenetic protein 2, IL-10, and leptin. The loss of function results in the failure of cells to respond appropriately to normal signaling.

There is a decrease in central memory (CD4- and CD8-positive T cells expressing CD27 and CD45RO) not due to apoptosis or cell turnover and stimulation of naive T cells with IL-7 or IL-15 failed to restore memory cell generation.[35] Defects in STAT3 decreases signaling through the T helper 1 pathway and skews toward T helper 2 cytokine production. Most cases are caused by de novo mutations.

Diagnosis

AD-HIES as a result of STAT3 dominant-negative mutations lead to eosinophilia and increased serum IgE. Often, the baseline increased total white blood cell count does not increase with acute infection. Neutropenia is rare, but has been reported, as have normal Ig levels. Numbers of T helper 17 cells assessed by flow cytometry or STAT3 phosphorylation are low. The gold standard is molecular diagnosis with sequencing of STAT3. Prenatal diagnosis is possible in familial STAT3 mutations.

Differential diagnosis

The HIES scoring system helps stratify the likelihood of a STAT3 mutation.[33] Other diseases should also be considered, including severe atopic dermatitis, cystic fibrosis, HIV, chronic granulomatous disease, and autosomal-recessive HIES (AR-HIES).

Management

Prevention and management of infections with long-term systemic antibiotics and antifungals is important. Lung abscesses may require operative intervention and aggressive management of possible complications. Although there is significant mortality, life expectancy can reach 50 years. Because some patients fail to sustain protective vaccination titers, Ig replacement should be initiated. HSCT is still under investigation, but has been used in severe disease.

Autosomal-Recessive Hyper-immunoglobulin E Syndrome

AR-HIES is also characterized by chronic eczema, recurrent staphylococcal skin infections, increased serum IgE, and peripheral blood eosinophilia. Clinically distinct from AD-HIES, these patients rarely have skeletal/dental abnormalities or coarse facial features. They are susceptible to severe viral infections (ie, herpes simplex virus, varicella zoster virus, and molluscum), and central nervous system manifestations (facial paralysis, hemiplegia, ischemic infarction, and subarachnoid hemorrhage), autoimmune diseases, and vascular disorders (aneurysms) are variably associated. Poor growth and failure to thrive is common. Unlike AD-HIES, 50% to 70% of patients develop severe allergies, including eczema, anaphylaxis to food, and environmental allergies, and 30% have asthma.[36] Pulmonary disease is usually asthma-related as compared with AD-HIES, where resulting pneumatocele and lung damage are the result of prior infections.

AR-HIES was originally described in 2004.[37] Most cases are caused by a defect in dedicator of the cytokinesis 8 (DOCK8) gene, and clinical features vary. In 2006, a defect in the signaling protein tyrosine kinase 2 (TYK2) was also identified as being inherited in an autosomal-recessive pattern.[38] Some support the classification of TYK2 homozygous mutation as a distinct atypical HIES with susceptibility to mycobacterium.[39] The prevalence of AR-HIES is less than 1 in 1,000,000[40] with some 130 affected families reported to date.

Pathogenesis
AR-HIES is a combined immune deficiency where DOCK8 or TYK2 mutations affect CD4 and CD8 proliferation, B cells, and memory cells. Homozygous mutations of DOCK8 (9p24.3) result in its loss of function. DOCK8 belongs to a subfamily of guanine nucleotide exchange factors, which have multiple roles, including signal transduction and activation of small G proteins. Recent evidence suggests that, although T and NK cells home and migrate into human tissue normally, the cytoskeletal defects in DOCK8-deficient T and NK cells lead to an unusual form of cell death—"cytothripsis" (cell shattering).[41] The inability of effector T cells and the absence of memory CD8+ T cells leave patients without protective immunity and a sensitivity to viral infection. Homozygous mutations in TYK2 (19p13) interrupt cytokine-controlled survival, proliferation, differentiation, and function of immune cells as well as others. This member of the JAK signaling family associates with the cytoplasmic domain of types 1 and 2 cytokines including interleukins, interferons, and hemopoietins by phosphorylating receptor subunits. Disruption of antiviral types 1 and 3 interferon signaling pathways lead to an increased susceptibility to viruses and mycobacterium.

Diagnosis
Similar to AD-HIES, AR-HIES patients have elevated total white blood cell counts that do not increase with acute infection, eosinophilia, and IgE. There are usually low T-cell numbers, low serum IgM levels, and a failure to sustain protective titers against vaccination. Owing to variability of presentation, flow cytometry for T helper 17 cells may be low. Clinically distinct features differentiate STAT3 AD-HIES and AR-HIES (DOCK8 and TYK2) mutations, which help to guide the appropriate genetic testing (see **Table 2**). The gold standard of diagnosis is molecular sequencing of these genes. Prenatal diagnosis should be considered if there is a family history.

Differential diagnosis
Other conditions to consider include severe eczema, AD-HIES, IPEX, HIV, Netherton syndrome, as well as SCID with skin graft versus host disease.

Management
Aggressive treatment of infection is critical to the care of patients with AR-HIES. The prognosis is poor, with most failing to reach adulthood as a result of sepsis, neurologic

disorders, and malignancies. Vascular complications (aneurysms) have been documented, including those secondary to vaccine-strain varicella zoster.[42] HSCT may be curative but remains experimental.

SUMMARY

The majority of patients with eczema, eosinophilia, and elevated IgE are likely to be atopic individuals that can be helped with some type of corticosteroid therapy. Oral corticosteroids have long been the mainstay of therapy to treat severe flares of allergic diseases. Direct binding of the glucocorticoid receptor complex to glucocorticoid responsive elements in the promoter region of genes, or by an interaction of this complex with other transcription factors such as activating protein-1 or nuclear factor-kappa-β inhibit production of many proinflammatory cytokines, chemokines, arachidonic acid metabolites, and adhesion molecules while concurrently upregulating anti-inflammatory mediators.[43] But, patients with the PIDs described rely on the remaining functioning parts of their immune system to control latent infections and combat opportunistic diseases (*Pneumocystis jirovecii*, *Mycobacterium avium* complex, and fungi). The broad scope of immune suppression by administered corticosteroids can lead to detrimental effects if an underlying PID goes unrecognized.[42,44,45] The increased risk (178-fold) of severe disseminated varicella infection owing to recent exposure to systemic corticosteroids[46] has been debated[47]; nevertheless, practitioners should exercise prudence before using elective systemic corticosteroids or other immune suppressants if there is a history of recurrent or opportunistic infection(s). Although highly effective and beneficial in otherwise healthy immune competent individuals with allergic flares, immune suppression of immune compromised PID individuals can lead to life-threatening dissemination of infection(s).[42,44]

PIDs are rare diseases that can be masked or not considered because of the predominant clinical features of atopy. Without considering an underlying PID, some individuals will remain undiagnosed and untreated, and this risk impacts their morbidity and mortality, especially when exposed to agents that further reduce immune competence. An underlying PID should be considered especially in severe cases of atopic disease with concurrent signs of autoimmunity and unusual infections so appropriate treatment regimens can be initiated and inappropriate immune suppression avoided.

REFERENCES

1. Rezaei N, Bonilla F, Sullivan K, et al. An introduction to primary immunodeficiency diseases. In: Rezaei N, Aghamohammadi A, Notarangelo L, editors. Primary Immunodeficiency Diseases: Definition, Diagnosis, Management. 5th edition. Berlin: Springer-Verlag; 2008. p. 1–38.
2. Boyle J, Buckley R. Population prevalence of diagnosed primary immunodeficiency diseases in the United States. J Clin Immunol 2007;27(5):497–502.
3. Pai S-Y, Logan BR, Griffith LM, et al. Transplantation outcomes for severe combined immunodeficiency, 2000-2009. N Engl J Med 2014;371(5):434–46.
4. Ozcan E, Notarangelo LD, Geha RS. Primary immune deficiencies with aberrant IgE production. J Allergy Clin Immunol 2008;122(6):1054–62 [quiz: 1063–4].
5. Laughter D, Istvan J, Tofte S, et al. The prevalence of atopic dermatitis in Oregon schoolchildren. J Am Acad Dermatol 2000;43(4):649–55.
6. Leung DY. Atopic dermatitis: the skin as a window into the pathogenesis of chronic allergic diseases. J Allergy Clin Immunol 1995;96(3):302–18 [quiz: 319].

7. Merithew E, Hatherly S, Dumas JJ, et al. Structural plasticity of an invariant hydrophobic triad in the switch regions of Rab GTPases is a determinant of effector recognition. J Biol Chem 2001;276(17):13982–8.

8. Rystedt I. Prognostic factors in atopic dermatitis. Acta Derm Venereol 1985;65(3):206–13.

9. Aleman K, Noordzij JG, de Groot R, et al. Reviewing Omenn syndrome. Eur J Pediatr 2001;160(12):718–25.

10. Omenn G. Familial reticuloendotheliosis with eosinophilia. N Engl J Med 1965;273:427–32.

11. Orpha.net. Omenn syndrome. Available at: www.orpha.net/consor/cgi-bin/Disease_Search.php?lng=EN&data_id=10452&Disease_Disease_Search_diseaseGroup=omen&Disease_Disease_Search_diseaseType=Pat&Disease%28s%29/group%20of%20diseases=Omenn-syndrome&title=Omenn-syndrome&search=Disease_Search_Simp. Accessed February 10, 2015.

12. Ege M, Ma Y, Manfras B, et al. Omenn syndrome due to ARTEMIS mutations. Blood 2005;105(11):4179–86.

13. Gomez L, Le Deist F, Blanche S, et al. Treatment of Omenn syndrome by bone marrow transplantation. J Pediatr 1995;127(1):76–81.

14. Powell BR, Buist NR, Stenzel P. An X-linked syndrome of diarrhea, polyendocrinopathy, and fatal infection in infancy. J Pediatr 1982;100(5):731–7.

15. Orpha.net. Immune dysregulation polyendocrinopathy enteropathy X-linked syndrome. Available at: www.orpha.net/consor/cgi-bin/Disease_Search.php?lng=EN&data_id=10440&Disease_Disease_Search_diseaseGroup=IPEX&Disease_Disease_Search_diseaseType=Pat&Disease%28s%29/group%20of%20diseases=Immune-dysregulation-polyendocrinopathy-enteropathy-X-linked-. Accessed February 10, 2015.

16. Ricciardelli I, Lindley KJ, Londei M, et al. Anti tumour necrosis-alpha therapy increases the number of FOXP3 regulatory T cells in children affected by Crohn's disease. Immunology 2008;125(2):178–83.

17. Van der Vliet HJJ, Nieuwenhuis EE. IPEX as a result of mutations in FOXP3. Clin Dev Immunol 2007;2007:89017.

18. Bindl L, Torgerson T, Perroni L, et al. Successful use of the new immune-suppressor sirolimus in IPEX (immune dysregulation, polyendocrinopathy, enteropathy, X-linked syndrome). J Pediatr 2005;147(2):256–9.

19. Baud O, Goulet O, Canioni D, et al. Treatment of the immune dysregulation, polyendocrinopathy, enteropathy, X-linked syndrome (IPEX) by allogeneic bone marrow transplantation. N Engl J Med 2001;344(23):1758–62.

20. Bacchetta R, Passerini L, Gambineri E, et al. Defective regulatory and effector T cell functions in patients with FOXP3 mutations. J Clin Invest 2006;116(6):1713–22.

21. Rao A, Kamani N, Filipovich A, et al. Successful bone marrow transplantation for IPEX syndrome after reduced-intensity conditioning. Blood 2007;109(1):383–5.

22. Aldrich R, Steinberg A, Campbell D. Pedigree demonstrating a sex-linked recessive condition characterized by draining ears, eczematoid dermatitis and bloody diarrhea. Pediatrics 1954;13(2):133–9.

23. Perry GS, Spector BD, Schuman LM, et al. The Wiskott-Aldrich syndrome in the United States and Canada (1892-1979). J Pediatr 1980;97(1):72–8.

24. Symons M, Derry JM, Karlak B, et al. Wiskott-Aldrich syndrome protein, a novel effector for the GTPase CDC42Hs, is implicated in actin polymerization. Cell 1996;84(5):723–34.

25. Simon HU, Mills GB, Hashimoto S, et al. Evidence for defective transmembrane signaling in B cells from patients with Wiskott-Aldrich syndrome. J Clin Invest 1992;90(4):1396–405.
26. Wada T, Schurman SH, Otsu M, et al. Somatic mosaicism in Wiskott-Aldrich syndrome suggests in vivo reversion by a DNA slippage mechanism. Proc Natl Acad Sci USA 2001;98(15):8697–702.
27. Boztug K, Germeshausen M, Avedillo Díez I, et al. Multiple independent second-site mutations in two siblings with somatic mosaicism for Wiskott-Aldrich syndrome. Clin Genet 2008;74(1):68–74.
28. Boztug K, Schmidt M, Schwarzer A, et al. Stem-cell gene therapy for the Wiskott-Aldrich syndrome. N Engl J Med 2010;363(20):1918–27.
29. Aiuti A, Biasco L, Scaramuzza S, et al. Lentiviral hematopoietic stem cell gene therapy in patients with Wiskott-Aldrich syndrome. Science 2013;341(6148):1233151.
30. Grimbacher B, Holland SM, Gallin JI, et al. Hyper-IgE syndrome with recurrent infections–an autosomal dominant multisystem disorder. N Engl J Med 1999; 340(9):692–702.
31. Davis SD, Schaller J, Wedgwood RJ. Job's Syndrome. Recurrent, "cold", staphylococcal abscesses. Lancet 1966;1(7445):1013–5.
32. Grimbacher B, Schäffer AA, Holland SM, et al. Genetic linkage of hyper-IgE syndrome to chromosome 4. Am J Hum Genet 1999;65(3):735–44.
33. Woellner C, Gertz EM, Schäffer AA, et al. Mutations in STAT3 and diagnostic guidelines for hyper-IgE syndrome. J Allergy Clin Immunol 2010;125(2): 424–32.e8.
34. Orpha.net. Autosomal dominant hyper-IgE syndrome. Available at: www.orpha.net/consor/cgi-bin/OC_Exp.php?Expert=2314&lng=EN. Accessed February 10, 2015.
35. Siegel AM, Heimall J, Freeman AF, et al. A critical role for STAT3 transcription factor signaling in the development and maintenance of human T cell memory. Immunity 2011;35(5):806–18.
36. Boos AC, Hagl B, Schlesinger A, et al. Atopic dermatitis, STAT3- and DOCK8-hyper-IgE syndromes differ in IgE-based sensitization pattern. Allergy 2014;69: 943–53.
37. Renner ED, Puck JM, Holland SM, et al. Autosomal recessive hyperimmunoglobulin E syndrome: a distinct disease entity. J Pediatr 2004;144(1):93–9.
38. Minegishi Y, Saito M, Morio T, et al. Human tyrosine kinase 2 deficiency reveals its requisite roles in multiple cytokine signals involved in innate and acquired immunity. Immunity 2006;25(5):745–55.
39. Woellner C, Schäffer AA, Puck JM, et al. The hyper IgE syndrome and mutations in TYK2. Immunity 2007;26(5):535 [author reply: 536].
40. Orpha.net. Autosomal recessive hyper-IgE syndrome. Available at: www.orpha. net/consor4.01/www/cgi-bin/Disease_Search.php?lng=EN&data_id=17857& Disease_Disease_Search_diseaseGroup=arHIES&Disease_Disease_Search_ diseaseType=Pat&Disease%28s%29/group%20of%20diseases=Autosomal-recessive-hyper-IgE-syndrome–AR-HIES-&tit. Accessed February 10, 2015.
41. Zhang Q, Dove C, Hor J, et al. DOCK8 regulates lymphocyte shape integrity for skin antiviral immunity. J Exp Med 2014;211(13):2549–66.
42. Sabry A, Hauk P, Jing H, et al. Vaccine strain varicella-zoster virus-induced central nervous system vasculopathy as the presenting feature of DOCK8 deficiency. J Allergy Clin Immunol 2014;133(4):1225–7.
43. Van der Velden V. Glucocorticoids: mechanisms of action and anti-inflammatory potential in asthma. Mediators Inflamm 1998;7(4):229–37.

44. Bayer DK, Seth N, Pearson N, et al. Atypical SCID with CD4 lymphopenia, hypergammaglobulinemi, and neutropenia presenting with disseminated vaccine-strain varicella and rubella infections. In: 2013 CIS Annual Meeting: Regulation & Dysregulation of Immunity. Miami, April 25–28, 2013.

45. Asai E, Wada T, Sakakibara Y, et al. Analysis of mutations and recombination activity in RAG-deficient patients. Clin Immunol 2011;138(2):172–7.

46. Dowell SF, Bresee JS. Severe varicella associated with steroid use. Pediatrics 1993;92(2):223–8.

47. Patel H. Recent corticosteroid use and the risk of complicated varicella in otherwise immunocompetent children. Arch Pediatr Adolesc Med 1996;150(4):409.

United States Postal Service
Statement of Ownership, Management, and Circulation
(All Periodicals Publications Except Requestor Publications)

1. Publication Title	2. Publication Number	3. Filing Date
Immunology and Allergy Clinics of North America	0 0 6 - 3 6 1	9/18/15

4. Issue Frequency	5. Number of Issues Published Annually	6. Annual Subscription Price
Feb, May, Aug, Nov	4	$320.00

7. Complete Mailing Address of Known Office of Publication (Not printer) (Street, city, county, state, and ZIP+4®)

Elsevier Inc.
360 Park Avenue South
New York, NY 10010-1710

Contact Person: Stephen R. Bushing
Telephone (Include area code): 215-239-3688

8. Complete Mailing Address of Headquarters or General Business Office of Publisher (Not printer)

Elsevier Inc., 360 Park Avenue South, New York, NY 10010-1710

9. Full Names and Complete Mailing Addresses of Publisher, Editor, and Managing Editor (Do not leave blank)

Publisher (Name and complete mailing address)

Linda Belfus, Elsevier Inc., 1600 John F. Kennedy Blvd., Suite 1800, Philadelphia, PA 19103

Editor (Name and complete mailing address)

Jessica McCool, Elsevier Inc., 1600 John F. Kennedy Blvd., Suite 1800, Philadelphia, PA 19103-2899

Managing Editor (Name and complete mailing address)

Adrianne Brigido, Elsevier Inc., 1600 John F. Kennedy Blvd., Suite 1800, Philadelphia, PA 19103-2899

10. Owner (Do not leave blank. If the publication is owned by a corporation, give the name and address of the corporation immediately followed by the names and addresses of all stockholders owning or holding 1 percent or more of the total amount of stock. If not owned by a corporation, give the names and addresses of the individual owners. If owned by a partnership or other unincorporated firm, give its name and address as well as those of each individual owner. If the publication is published by a nonprofit organization, give its name and address.)

Full Name	Complete Mailing Address
Wholly owned subsidiary of	1600 John F. Kennedy Blvd, Ste. 1800
Reed/Elsevier, US holdings	Philadelphia, PA 19103-2899

11. Known Bondholders, Mortgagees, and Other Security Holders Owning or Holding 1 Percent or More of Total Amount of Bonds, Mortgages, or Other Securities. If none, check box ☐ None

Full Name	Complete Mailing Address
N/A	

12. Tax Status (For completion by nonprofit organizations authorized to mail at nonprofit rates) (Check one)
The purpose, function, and nonprofit status of this organization and the exempt status for federal income tax purposes:
☐ Has Not Changed During Preceding 12 Months
☐ Has Changed During Preceding 12 Months (Publisher must submit explanation of change with this statement)

13. Publication Title	14. Issue Date for Circulation Data Below
Immunology and Allergy Clinics of North America	August 2015

15. Extent and Nature of Circulation			Average No. Copies Each Issue During Preceding 12 Months	No. Copies of Single Issue Published Nearest to Filing Date
a. Total Number of Copies (Net press run)			393	309
b. Legitimate Paid and/Or Requested Distribution (By Mail and Outside the Mail)	(1)	Mailed Outside-County Paid/Requested Mail Subscriptions stated on PS Form 3541. (Include paid distribution above nominal rate, advertiser's proof copies and exchange copies)	200	160
	(2)	Mailed In-County Paid/Requested Mail Subscriptions stated on PS Form 3541. (Include paid distribution above nominal rate, advertiser's proof copies and exchange copies)		
	(3)	Paid Distribution Outside the Mails Including Sales Through Dealers And Carriers, Street Vendors, Counter Sales, and Other Paid Distribution Outside USPS®	43	54
	(4)	Paid Distribution by Other Classes of Mail Through the USPS (e.g. First-Class Mail®)		
c. Total Paid and or Requested Circulation (Sum of 15b (1), (2), (3), and (4))			243	214
d. Free or Nominal Rate Distribution (By Mail and Outside the Mail)	(1)	Free or Nominal Rate Outside-County Copies included on PS Form 3541	60	33
	(2)	Free or Nominal Rate In-County Copies included on PS Form 3541		
	(3)	Free or Nominal Rate Copies mailed at Other classes Through the USPS (e.g. First-Class Mail®)		
	(4)	Free or Nominal Rate Distribution Outside the Mail (Carriers or Other means)		
e. Total Nonrequested Distribution (Sum of 15d (1), (2), (3) and (4)			60	33
f. Total Distribution (Sum of 15c and 15e)			303	247
g. Copies not Distributed (See instructions to publishers #4 (page #3))			90	62
h. Total (Sum of 15f and g)			393	309
i. Percent Paid and/or Requested Circulation (15c divided by 15f times 100)			80.20%	86.64%

* If you are claiming electronic copies go to line 16 on page 3. If you are not claiming Electronic copies, skip to line 17 on page 3.

16. Electronic Copy Circulation	Average No. Copies Each Issue During Preceding 12 Months	No. Copies of Single Issue Published Nearest to Filing Date
a. Paid Electronic Copies		
b. Total paid Print Copies (Line 15c) + Paid Electronic Copies (Line 16a)		
c. Total Print Distribution (Line 15f) + Paid Electronic Copies (Line 16a)		
d. Percent Paid (Both Print & Electronic copies) (16b divided by 16c X 100)		

☐ I certify that 50% of all my distributed copies (electronic and print) are paid above a nominal price

17. Publication of Statement of Ownership
☐ If the publication is a general publication, publication of this statement is required. Will be printed in the **November 2015** issue of this publication.

18. Signature and Title of Editor, Publisher, Business Manager, or Owner

Stephen R. Bushing — Stephen R. Bushing Inventory Distribution Coordinator

Date: September 18, 2015

I certify that all information furnished on this form is true and complete. I understand that anyone who furnishes false or misleading information on this form or who omits material or information requested on the form may be subject to criminal sanctions (including fines and imprisonment) and/or civil sanctions (including civil penalties).

PS Form 3526, July 2014 (Page 1 of 3 (Instructions Page 3)) PSN 7530-01-000-9931 PRIVACY NOTICE: See our Privacy policy in www.usps.com

PS Form 3526, July 2014 (Page 2 of 3)

PS Form 3526, July 2014 (Page 3 of 3)

Printed and bound by CPI Group (UK) Ltd, Croydon, CR0 4YY

03/10/2024

01040492-0017